CANCER SUCKS

A True Story

CANCER SUCKS

A True Story

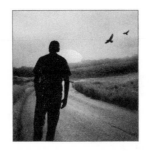

DAVID YATES

one man's journey

Two Harbors Press

Minneapolis, MN

Two Harbors Press
212 3rd Avenue North, Suite 290
Minneapolis, MN 55401
612.455.2293
www.TwoHarborsPress.com

The information in this book is based on a true story. The names of some people, descriptions, and places have been changed to protect identities. The location could be any and/or all cities and towns throughout America, as well as other countries. This book is for those living with cancer, facing cancer surgery and chemotherapy, and for those incredible individuals who take care of us.

This book is not intended to replace, supplement, or conflict with the advice of your personal physician, cancer specialists, or cancer hospitals and institutes. My recommendation is to follow your doctor's advice, but never be afraid to ask questions. After all, it is your life.

The author disclaims any and all liability with the use of this book.

ISBN-13: 978-1-936401-94-9
LCCN: 2011930325

Distributed by Itasca Books

Cover Design and Typeset by Sophie Chi

Printed in the United States of America

DEDICATION

This book is dedicated to everyone who is a statistic of cancer, to those who currently have cancer, and to cancer survivors.

Thanks to all of our caregivers, past and present; doctors, nurses, hospitals, family, friends; and to all cancer foundations, institutes, and camps. Without you, our challenges and recovery would be impossible.

TABLE OF CONTENTS

FOREWORD

David's story is moving and inspiring. It underlines the importance of mental strength and a good support network for cancer patients, as well as the crucial importance that we in the medical community continue to improve our scientific understanding of this highly complex "disease." As a cancer researcher in the pharmaceutical industry, stories like David's motivate me to invent better therapies that will benefit future cancer patients. For many of us working in the cancer pharmaceutical industry, our motivation is often personal. We've had family members or close friends who have had cancer, too.

There is clearly a need for more effective treatments with better side effect profiles for all types of cancer. For many patients there are no effective drugs that can treat their tumors, or the best drugs currently available are merely palliative in that they aim to improve the patient's quality of life rather than survival. David's portacath experience (chapter 14) also shows that how we administer the drug can make a real difference to patients' well-being and the success of the treatment. Our success so far has been limited by the complexity of cancer. In reality, cancer is not a single disease; even within colon cancer, the cause of the tumor growth will vary from patient to patient, and thus how the tumor will respond to chemotherapy may be unpredictable for novel treatments or new combinations of existing treatments. Dr. Rosen's decision to avoid combining the "magic mushrooms" with David's chemotherapy (chapter 8) might seem harsh but is understandable given the lack of information she had to say whether this combination would benefit David.

Cancer does indeed suck, but I'm constantly awed by the personal bravery of cancer sufferers and their loved ones, and by the professionalism and dedication of those who work to improve the lives of cancer patients. As a scientist, I'm encouraged by the speed at which scientists are improving our understanding of this highly complex disease, and I'm optimistic that the treatments we discover in the future will continue to improve people's lives. As David says, we should never give up!

Dr. Frederick Goldberg, oncology researcher [1]

---

[1] Dr. Frederick Goldberg works for AstraZeneca, but this foreword has been written in a personal capacity. The views expressed are his own.

PROLOGUE

CANCER SUCKS!

BULLETS SPRAYED the mud around me and pinged off a disabled fire truck thirty feet away. I slid into a trench parallel to a chain-link fence in our compound that was in serious danger of being overrun by the Viet Cong. I held my breath each time I heard an incoming mortar, but then I realized that as long as I heard the explosion, I was still alive. Then, two Cobra gunships (attack helicopters loaded with machine guns and rockets that had a distinct spine-chilling growl) came from out of nowhere and drove back the VC. I was as terrified as I had ever been in my life, wondering if I would ever make it home to see my family.

The Vietnam War was filled with horror and death just like any other war, and it left thousands of soldiers with injuries and diseases: cancer was just one of many. I was one of the lucky ones; my cancer was detected while I was still in the Army. Others weren't so fortunate; their problems weren't discovered until after they left the military, so they were left to face the financial and physical trauma alone. Sometimes I feel guilty because I was medically taken care of by the military and the Veteran's Administration while others weren't. I wish I knew then what I know now—perhaps I could have made a difference in someone's life—but what does a twenty-one-year-old know in 1968? Though there is probably nothing I can ever do for the soldiers of the Vietnam War, perhaps some will find solace reading this. I owe them my gratitude, just as all of us owe gratitude to those presently fighting around the world to keep America free.

There are many forms of fear and anxiety; war is near the top of my list, and there are numerous situations and visions of war I will never forget. Those memories are something I live with, just like all soldiers returning from war. But Vietnam and all of its horrors didn't even come a close second to the anxiety I experienced when faced with cancer, surgery, and chemotherapy. That's why I will never end my personal war against cancer. I believe with all of my heart that one way or the other, we will defeat this enemy. Whether it is accomplished by all of humanity, our culture, or other cultures, cancer will one day be known only by looking back and studying history. Obliteration, eradication, and annihilation are words that will be used to describe the disappearance of this once-humbling disease. But that time is unknown, much like the unknown most of us face when experiencing cancer and chemotherapy, and perhaps I will not live to see that day, but the contribution we make as individuals, or as an entity, can and will be beneficial to the future generation that claims the ultimate victory over this dreaded enemy. After all, it is the number one killer in the world.

The devastating effects of cancer are often overshadowed when compared to heart attacks, strokes, diseases with physical maladies (i.e., muscular dystrophy and multiple sclerosis), and the unfathomable list of motives, such as loneliness and depression, as to why anyone would choose to give up on life. However, coupled with chemotherapy and/or radiation, the effects of cancer should be CAPITALIZED and set in **BOLD** type, much like flashing neon signs on the Vegas strip. Together, although both operate under the disguise of curative, cancer and chemotherapy are co-assassins that work to strip an individual of the will to live—an instinct that is deeply rooted within each and every soul awaiting the trumpeting call from a higher power.

Life is amazingly precious, and I've always thought of myself as strong and unrelenting and a sound representative of humanity who would never adopt a quitting attitude. But I readily admit that at times when the reality of sickness became overwhelming I, too, (though briefly) entertained thoughts of "giving up" or "checking out." But somehow I was able to banish that alternative to the darkest caverns of my mind. I love life. The beauty in the world around us is oftentimes breathtaking, and giving in, to me, would be much the same as committing suicide—I refused to go there.

I do not, and will not, judge or second-guess anyone's right or decision to abandon ship in the often stormy waters of an ill-fated voyage with cancer—it is a God-given choice—but I am an individual spirit and must always answer to my inner soul.

I've battled cancer three times in my life: twice with malignant melanoma and once with a tumor of the cecum. Each case was not only physically and emotionally damaging but also draining on my spirit. However, I firmly believe that the spirit rules, and, depending on where and how we are spiritually aligned, if we allow our spirits to govern, we can conquer anything.

With each cancerous battle, I did not associate dying with the disease, at least not at that particular time. I chose instead to call those battles life challenges. Whether or not that made a difference to my survival, I accept the fact that one day it will likely be cancer that ultimately destroys my physical body and claims my life on this earth. But it can never consume my soul or who I am.

Who am I?

I'm David Yates from Santa Domingo, California: husband, father, friend, and lover of life. I am sixty-three years of age, six feet three inches tall, and 235 pounds. With reddish-blonde hair now laced with white, I'm an English, Scottish, Irish mix, and from my father's heritage, perhaps one-quarter Cherokee Indian. But more than that, I am an American, of which I am enormously proud.

But nationality is insignificant when it comes to cancer. This disease is one of the few that does not discriminate. It cares not about race, gender, sexual and political preference, or religion. Young or old does not matter, nor whether a person is tall and thin or short and fat. Cancer does not give a damn who it attacks. Wealthy or poor, we are all subject to the potential destruction of this silent killer.

Even the healthiest of individuals fall victim to cancer—as if cancer's sole purpose is to inflict turmoil upon a seemingly normal life. Whether bodybuilder or bookworm, athlete or couch potato, blue-collar or white-collar worker, smoker or non-smoker, educated or unlearned, Democrat,

Independent, or Republican, rich or poor, we are all potential prey.

My time on this earth will one day end, but until then I will continue to fight all cancer-related obstacles with every ounce of my being and I will enjoy every God-given breath to its fullest. My hope is that everyone who reads this book will join me in never giving up. You can do it. Sure, it's hard to stay positive and keep going day after day when cancer never takes a break—the disease is relentless and pursues us until our final breath—but we must never give up.

Every breath we take beyond our expectations is a small victory, and as those victories multiply, so do our chances of wiping this killer off the face of the earth. More than anything, I want to live to see that day and celebrate with the world, rejoicing with those who have cancer and for those who were forced to let go.

One way or the other, we are destined to win this battle. We will not give up. We will not quit.

CHAPTER 1

Cancer for the Third Time

Round One

IT WAS unseasonably warm for mid-November in 1968 at Fort Gordon, Georgia. I had been back in the United States for seven months after a demoralizing year in Vietnam. The dress code was summer khakis, our Army field jackets were still in boxes.

I was twenty-one at the time and married—my first child was born while I was in Vietnam, something I regret to this day. (It's not easy being away from your wife and family when your child is born, but I love my country and would do it again in an instant.)

I remember the day with clarity, as though it just happened. A seasoned supply sergeant major I worked for noticed blood on the white T-shirt beneath my starched fatigue collar. He was considered a grouchy lifer by those who knew him, and he appeared much older than his fifty-five years, yet he reminded me of my grandfather. He was six feet tall and solidly built with a face heavily wrinkled from years of exposure to the sun. His skin was as rough as cowhide and his forearms were as thick as oak branches. Despite his demanding character, I knew him to have a compassionate heart and to be as kind as a summer day is long. After noticing the mole on my neck and the bloody chain clipped to my dog tags, he barked orders, referring me to the base hospital. "Yates!" he bellowed, "get your ass to the hospital." Call it luck of the draw, life, or destiny, but there is little doubt that he was one of many uniquely stationed in my life for a particular purpose.

As far as I knew, the distorted mole on my neck was nothing out of the ordinary; it had begun to bleed earlier that year while in Vietnam from the constant irritation of towel drying, dog tags, and fatigue collars. I recall a gung ho second lieutenant in our compound who saddled me with additional guard duty because of the embedded blood splotches on my collars. (The mama-sans who did our laundry did the best they could, but blood stains are hard to get out.) I wanted to remind him that we were in a battle zone and that blood on fatigues was a common sight, but my protests would likely have been labeled insubordination and perhaps resulted in a court martial. (As I learned soon after arriving in Vietnam, second lieutenants fresh out of West Point were not only gung ho, but most of them also operated strictly from military manuals and textbooks; they were slow to look at a situation logically. Thank God for the non-commissioned officers.)

At the hospital, I met with a flamboyant young surgeon: a short, red-haired captain from New York. He was serving a two-year commitment after negotiating government funds for medical school, and he, too, was immediately alarmed by the mole. He ordered a biopsy, and a few days later I learned the results.

The diagnosis? Malignant melanoma. It was considered stage "3-C" (the label "3-C" was given after the operation and from the results of the lab tests), which means the cancer involved more than three lymph nodes but it was uncertain whether there was further metastasis.

The cause? Unknown; although, after conversations with several physicians, Agent Orange—the code name for an herbicide and defoliant used by the United States Military in its Herbicidal Warfare program during the Vietnam War—appeared the most likely culprit. The government denied spraying the deadly chemical in the area of Vietnam where I was stationed just as they once denied our presence in Cambodia. To this day, those who make the policy decisions still refuse to link Agent Orange with melanoma and colon cancer. Most dermatologists emphatically claim that melanomas are only caused by ultraviolet rays that damage a cell's DNA, but other physicians and chiropractors agree that chemicals can cause the disease.

The procedure? Right radical neck dissection, which included removal of neck tissue, sternocleidomastoid muscle, lymph nodes, and saliva glands. Because of the contaminated lymph nodes and saliva glands, the possibility of metastasis was high, but the doctors were not sure what would happen.

The prognosis? Wait and see. If I was lucky, I would survive. If not, I would be another causality of cancer (not the Vietnam War) and most likely be dead within a year. I was told that melanomas were not radiation-sensitive, so that procedure would have little or no effect. And chemotherapy at the time was evidently not an option.

The recovery from surgery was extensive—a drain tube was left in the incision area to prevent infection and skin grafts and considerable physical therapy were necessary due to the limited range of motion in my shoulder. My mental and emotional recovery was also lengthy—I had to process the fact that I would never live out my boyhood dream of playing professional baseball.

I've always loved sports, but baseball was my favorite. I learned to throw a ball when I was knee-high to a billy goat. I was always tall for my age and oftentimes intimidating as a pitcher. At age twelve, in 1960, I struck out every hitter that came to the plate in a Little League game. During American Legion baseball (Palm Beach Post 12) after my senior year at Forest Hill High

School in 1965, I was invited by a scout to try out for the Los Angeles Dodgers at their spring training facility in Vero Beach, Florida. During American Legion baseball in 1966, the Cincinnati Reds were interested, but so was Uncle Sam. And I quickly learned that Uncle Sam gets what he wants.

Did I feel cheated? Absolutely. Cancer had decided not to kill me but to rob me of what I loved most in life: baseball. Cancer really does suck. At that moment, it not only became my enemy, but I declared war against it. I also knew it was going to be a tougher and longer battle than the Vietnam War.

Round Two

Twenty-one months later—I was a civilian then and medically followed by the Veteran's Administration Hospital in Miami, Florida—a knot the size of an extra-large egg in the same area of my neck told me that the cancer had returned. I was devastated. I had no idea what I was going to do. Without a personal physician, without a support group or friends who knew anything about cancer to advise me, I had only those at the VA and my wife and three-year-old son to whom I could talk and entrust my life. So that's exactly what I did. The doctors and nurses at the VA proved to be professional and friendly, and I felt as comfortable with them as I did with family. (There was a great deal of waiting involved with each checkup and hospital stay at the VA and I was mostly referred to by a number, but the government was the only insurance I had. I'm lucky and thankful they took care of me.)

The diagnosis? A biopsy revealed the reoccurrence of malignant melanoma. (It seemed as though I couldn't get rid of this persistent enemy.)

The cause? Renegade malignant cells from the original surgery. It didn't matter if the reoccurrence was due to the surgery dispersing the tumor cells or if the cancer was more involved than originally suspected, it was back.

The procedure? Additional surgery to remove the tumor, surrounding tissue, and those lymph nodes left after the initial surgery.

The prognosis? The fact that the cancer had returned was strong evidence that the malignancy had metastasized. Not good; I had maybe three to six months to live.

Physical recovery from the second surgery was much faster, except for another skin graft, but the emotional challenge was, at times, more than I thought I could handle. Once again, neither chemotherapy nor radiation was offered as an option.

The thought of having only three to six months to live was pretty frightening, but when I recalled my "Declaration of War" against my adversary and the fact that my wife was pregnant, it gave me renewed strength. More than anything I wanted to live long enough to see the birth of my second child.

As I said before, I never once thought I was going to die. Why? Maybe at age twenty-two I was too mean and stubborn to allow cancer to win—I wasn't too different from the naive twenty-year-old I had been in a firefight in Vietnam determined that I was invincible and that dying was what happened to others. After all, I wasn't afraid to die. I was more afraid of the unknowns of living with my adversary. Perhaps I was just plain lucky, or maybe the surgeons were completely wrong about the extent of the disease. Whatever the reason, I am thankful to be alive. As I have aged, I am more and more convinced that my survival has everything to do with my spiritual nature and my desire and ability to fight. So fight I did.

I decided to live my life as if I had already survived cancer instead of sitting around waiting to die—an attitude that was instilled in me at a very young age by my mother. Whether it was sports (baseball or basketball), music (the marching band in seventh grade at Vero Beach High School), youth programs at church, or anything else I wanted to do, it was forbidden to quit once I had begun. And she was always with me at every game. She supported and encouraged me when I won and comforted me when I lost. She taught me to win and lose graciously and to always be aware of others' feelings. But the one thing that she insisted on was that I fight for what I wanted. I remember her words as if she had just spoken them to me: "Nothing is out of your grasp. If you believe in something, fight for it with all of your heart. If you fail at something, get back up and do it again. And do not quit!"

So my young family (which now included two small children) and I took off for Baton Rouge and LSU, Louisiana State University.

If I could no longer play baseball, I wanted to be an architect, but I settled for a degree in General Education with a concentration in sociology and psychology.

During my life at LSU—an incredible academic and athletic school—I was followed yearly on an outpatient basis by the VA Hospital in New Orleans. Each year my checkup was clean: no cancer. (I was even involved in a personal two-week study at the VA Medical Center in New Orleans that researched why I hadn't died. The physicians put me through numerous tests they hoped would produce results to explain my miraculous recovery. But they found nothing to answer their questions. And here I am, still alive.)

By the time I graduated from LSU in 1975, I had been cancer free, or in remission, for almost five years. I had beaten the odds for a five-year survival and I was grateful, but the reality that cancer could return at any time was always looming like a dark cloud. I'm reminded every day when I look at my scars in the mirror of what might have been, but my self-pity is short-lived because I am truly thankful to be alive.

As the years passed, my third child was born. My architecture experience at LSU proved beneficial, and I chose the construction industry as a profession. I decided that I would rather build a structure than design it.

My health was good. Life was good. And there was still no sign of cancer.

Then, in 1989 (after twenty-three years of marriage and three children—David, DeAunna, and Daryl—the unthinkable happened: a divorce. I've always believed that when I married it was for better or worse, and that it was forever. Sure, it does take two to make a marriage successful, and it takes a lot of work, but sometimes bad things just happen. I needed a change, so "Southern California here I come."

Needless to say, I didn't have much confidence in women at this time. In fact, on my drive to California, I made a list of ten traits and qualities that the next woman I allowed into my life had to possess. Impossible to find, right? Maybe, but little did I know it would only take three weeks to find the one who possessed nine of the ten qualities I had listed. I wasn't even looking for a new relationship. But sometimes good things just happen. It was unquestionably love at first sight. I knew she was my soul mate: Debbie. She had a three-year-old daughter, Amanda, when we met. And, yes, being a mother was on the list.

Sixteen years with Debbie and Amanda passed quickly. Life was again good. We were all healthy and I had been cancer-free for almost thirty-six years, until that dreadful phone call from my primary care physician.

Round Three

"David, this is Dr. Stone."

I've only had one other phone call from a physician—when my father died fourteen years ago. I was completely dumbfounded. "Hello, Dr. Stone. My physical isn't until Friday."

"I just reviewed the results of your blood test. I want to see you in my office as soon as possible."

It was one thirty Monday afternoon in late July, 2006, and I didn't want to make an unnecessary trip to Conchita, a small town about fifteen miles east of Santa Domingo.

"Can't it wait until Friday? I can come in a little early if you'd like."

Dr. Stone was direct. "I would like to see you right away."

I was suddenly worried. "What's wrong?"

"I'll save that for when you get here."

"I'll be there in half an hour."

I had passed dumbfounded and was approaching shock as I drove the freeway to Dr. Stone's office, thoughts swarming in my head like a hive of angry bees. I couldn't imagine what was so urgent that couldn't wait until Friday. Maybe I was in the beginning stages of diabetes, or perhaps my cholesterol was seriously high. Anemia crossed my mind, as did a sluggish thyroid or a bacterial infection, but they were abnormalities that could wait until my physical on Friday, weren't they?

I signed in at the receptionist window, and then I sat in the packed waiting room for only three minutes (perhaps the shortest wait in recorded history to see a physician) before I was ushered past angry patients into Dr. Stone's cramped office.

We shook hands and I sat in the only chair in front of his desk. He was average height, energetic, and middle-aged with a boyish face and compassionate blue eyes. There was an air of confidence about him that eased the blood pressure of most of his patients, including, at the moment, mine. He directed my attention to a list of test results—most of which were in the normal to good range. However, he explained that my red blood cell count was 7.7, a dangerously low number when compared to normal levels between fourteen and eighteen.

"What does that mean?" I asked.

"It means you're losing blood, a lot of it."

The revelation further calmed me. I had been diagnosed with diverticulitis several years earlier after an emergency room visit for abdominal pain. At the time, I presumed it to be a kidney stone, but a stool sample and CT scan revealed diverticulitis: inflammation of pouches, or diverticula, that had formed in the large intestine. And then I recalled the reason I had scheduled the upcoming physical examination: a very bloody stool and acute fatigue. "It must be the diverticulitis acting up again," I said. "I have a confession to make," and then I paused, "I haven't been all that faithful to the diet you prescribed."

"It could be diverticulitis, or a number of other things," replied Dr. Stone, "but I want you to have a colonoscopy and an upper endoscopy. That's the only way we'll know for sure."

"You think that's really necessary?" I asked.

"Very."

Three days later I was sitting in an examining room at Dr. Thomas Sparrow's office, a general surgeon and friend of Dr. Stone's in Conchita. The visit with Dr. Sparrow lasted almost an hour and consisted mostly of family and personal history. By the time I left his office, I was scheduled for the colonoscopy and upper endoscopy the following Monday.

I certainly wasn't looking forward to it, but the colonoscopy literally saved my life. And it was as easy as passing gas, seriously. The only discomfort was drinking the bowel cleansing solution to cleanse my system prior to the procedure. It's not the most pleasant tasting liquid to drink (my taste buds described it as a mixture of ocean water and castor oil), but it certainly did the job.

And it's a must to go into a colonoscopy with a clean colon. With each subsequent colonoscopy I tried to mask the taste with other drinks like Gatorade, grape juice, and any other type of clear liquid I could think of that would mask the taste. It helped somewhat, but it also increased the amount of liquid I had to consume and prolonged the effectiveness time. Regardless of how you choose to drink the solution, I would not plan activity away from the house. Within a short period of time, the porcelain god will be your friend.

As with any invasive procedure, there can be a downside to a colonoscopy. Roughly one-third of one percent of those undergoing a colonoscopy have some difficulty. There is the possibility of perforation to the colon necessitating surgery to remove a portion of the colon. Please make sure you have a qualified gastroenterologist performing the procedure. And don't be afraid to ask the physician as many questions as you wish. It is your colon— your body—your life.

But even with the minute risk involved, a colonoscopy is normally a safe procedure.

To say I was a little nervous is like saying a woman is a little pregnant, and, to make matters worse, I had suffered from panic attacks over the past five years. One psychologist believed them to be caused by Post Traumatic Stress Disorder, or PTSD, possibly related to the horrors of the Vietnam War. Dr. Sparrow knew about my anxiety from the consultation in his office and left orders for the pre-op nurses at the same-day surgery clinic at University Hospital to administer Ativan as soon as they started the IV. By the time Dr. Sparrow arrived at the hospital for the procedure, I was as relaxed as a hibernating bear.

Though I was foggy after the Ativan, I knew. I've always been an eternal optimist and look for the good in people and life. I believe that mind can overrule matter, but I also know when to call a spade a spade. But it wasn't until later that afternoon when I awoke on the couch at home that I truly understood the words Dr. Sparrow had spoken to Debbie: "I'm so sorry to have to tell you this, but your husband has colon cancer."

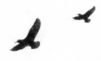

CHAPTER 2

Coming to Terms

THE FOLLOWING three days were incomprehensible. I couldn't believe that my old enemy had returned and that the war was still on. I often felt as if I were trapped in a realm somewhere between this world and the next, where a frightening dream suddenly turns real. It was a shock to my total being to realize that I had cancer again (the lab results indicated that the biopsy was highly suspicious). According to Dr. Sparrow, surgery was the best option. He had seen it hundreds of times. He knew, and I knew.

I wrestled emotionally with the stages of grief, especially denial, anger, and depression. I hate to cry (I was taught by my father at an early age that men don't cry), but it felt good to get it out. But then I would deny it was happening to me. Someone else's tests had gotten mixed up with mine.

That was it—a hospital error. I'd been too healthy throughout my life, except for the previous two cancers and a few kidney stones. My daily diet consisted of all of the food groups, though sometimes I consumed more red meat than recommended, and sports and exercise had always been an integral part of my daily regimen. So, this could not be happening to me. But the more I rationalized the more I understood that a good diet and exercise program are not enough. Checkups and physical exams are equally important to remaining healthy. Admitting my shortcomings in this area was overwhelming. I wondered if I wanted to go on, or why I should go on. After all, cancer had already robbed me of my boyhood dream of playing pro baseball and forced me into a life I hadn't planned on living. Why not just give in and get it over with? I decided to make a list of "why I should" and "why I shouldn't." I didn't get very far because the first "why I should" was my mother's maxim: Do Not Quit! The second "why I should" was Debbie, and she was enough to make anyone want to live.

I didn't even entertain thoughts of the third stage, bargaining, because I don't believe it's fair to make promises to a higher power I know I most likely will not keep. I've heard friends and family pray to survive a particular operation, disease, or even something as trivial as winning a ballgame, for which they solemnly vowed to change their lives by giving to and helping others, if only HE would grant their prayer. In all cases the promises were short-lived and they were back to their old habits (hate your neighbor but don't forget to say grace).

Then I was angry, angry at cancer and the scientists for not finding a cure, angry at all of the companies and their employees who make products that are harmful to the environment and our bodies and can cause cancer, and I was angry at humanity for buying those products. I was angry at the government for making me fight in a war and exposing me to Agent Orange. I was angry at everyone and everything. And when I was finished being angry at others, I was angry with myself for neglecting my body.

I came to terms with anger, at least I thought I did, and I felt better. But then I was depressed. I felt like being alone much of the time. I was listless and often felt as though I was living in slow motion. However, there are no distinct lines separating the stages of grief. I bounced from anger to depression and back again without understanding why. And then it would begin again.

I even asked all the relative questions, the most frequent being, "Why me, God? Why do I have to go through this again? Haven't I had my share of sickness and trauma? Isn't it someone else's turn?" But I knew the answer.

Accepting the blame for our actions is not always easy. It is much simpler to put it on someone else, even God. But I believe with all my heart that God has no hand or joy in seeing that which He created suffer. We are given free will to make our own choices in life, and we are at our present station because of those decisions. But once we accept the fact that we are the authors of the life challenges we face, our spirits overpower our egos and create a fight within us that we had no idea even existed.

I had ignored the advice of my doctor, friends, and my adorable wife, Debbie, for over seven years about having a colonoscopy.

"I don't need a colonoscopy," I had insisted each time the subject surfaced. "I eliminate after every meal, so how could I have something growing inside of me?"

I found out the hard way that the number of daily eliminations is not relevant when speaking of colon cancer. But there was another reason I did not want a colonoscopy.

I've had numerous experiences in hospitals that were far too unpleasant, and I wanted nothing more to do with smells of antiseptic and death. The most terrifying event I could think of, after a disastrous recovery-room incident after kidney stones four years earlier, which induced my first panic attack, was putting my trust in another anesthesiologist. I was wrong. As a Monday morning quarterback, I now know how easy it is to endure a colonoscopy, and if I had known just how easy it was, I would have consented years ago. In fact, I'm the only one I know who is looking forward to the next one. My hope is that anyone reading this book who is over fifty (or those younger with a family history of colon cancer) will not procrastinate; please, have it done. It could save you and your loved ones a great deal of pain and suffering.

I can't express in words how important it is to have someone in your life to help you through the stages of grief. I don't think there can be a substitute for kindness, care, and love from another human being when faced with cancer. That's why I can't write another word without telling you about Debbie. She is kind and compassionate and as beautiful on the inside as she is physically. Energy radiates through her like an adrenalin high. But it was her eyes—the color of a turquoise bay in the Caribbean—and her Wisconsin-Cheesehead smile that first attracted me; the same warm smile that normally accompanies those in a service profession who are kind and caring and spend most of their lives helping others. Without a doubt she is my rock and the wind in my sail, and she is the main reason I'm still living and functioning on this earth. She has more patience in her little finger than I do in my entire body. She was efficient in the way she took charge of the situation—the beginning and end, alpha and omega—and in the way she took care of me. She encouraged me through good and difficult days. She suffered with me, but she remained strong and held my hand during the entire journey. I'm thankful I had her, and I hope that those with cancer enduring chemotherapy and/or radiation, or any other disease or physical anomaly, have a Debbie. I can't imagine having survived without her, or even wanting to.

It was Debbie's encouragement that led me to the last stage of grief: acceptance.

I was determined to continue my war with cancer and grow old with Debbie. Acceptance doesn't mean that everything is going to be okay or that life will be the same as it was before cancer, but it does mean accepting the life challenge and moving in a positive direction.

Change is inevitable, and it is how we handle that change that defines who we want to be and who we are. Perhaps life will never be the same, but it can be as good as we want it to be. "You have cancer," Debbie said, "now let's get rid of it."

Debbie and I made the decision together to fight this frightening disease with all of our joined heart and soul. No negative thoughts, ever (yes, it's definitely easier to say than to do). I knew if I was going to survive, I had to remain in control of my life.

Debbie held my hand the following Tuesday as we sat in one of Dr. Sparrow's examining rooms. When he entered, his confidence and kindness leading the way, he sat on a rolling stool in front of us. He was heavier and older than Dr. Stone by at least fifteen years with a 1950s crew cut the color of a silver fox.

"How are you feeling?" he asked.

"Good, but tired," I replied.

"I would expect that," he said. "Due to your low red blood count, I'm surprised you're not sleeping all day. That's the first thing we need to take care of."

"How do we do that?" Debbie asked.

"We do that with a blood transfusion. He needs to be stronger for the operation, which I've scheduled for a week from Thursday."

"A blood transfusion is necessary?" I asked.

"Absolutely," Dr. Sparrow said.

He saw the concern on my face and assured me that in this day and age, getting struck by lightning was far more likely than getting a disease from tainted blood. His words were reassuring, and I trusted him completely.

We asked him, after a hundred other questions, if we should wait a few weeks after the transfusion to make sure I was strong enough. He answered, "Would you wait to remove a rotten apple until it had infected the entire barrel?"

Satisfied with his answer, we also asked if there were new drugs and therapy used in clinical trials that were not yet on the market from which I could benefit.

"There are always studies in progress with new drugs and procedures," he said, "and I'm sure we could find one for you if it were really necessary. But I don't think your case warrants this process. I think surgery is the best answer here, and possibly a follow-up with chemotherapy."

"How long is the operation?" Debbie asked.

"Surgery such as this usually takes about three hours, depending on what I find," Dr. Sparrow said. And then he explained that he would take out the diseased portion of my colon, surrounding tissue, and lymph nodes for testing. "Under normal conditions," he continued, "I expect to remove eight to twelve inches of colon. And in this case, I doubt an ostomy bag will be necessary."

I nodded as if I understood, yet there was no way for me to realize the extent of what was going to happen. So, my apprehension continued, and two days later I was hooked to an IV in a small room in the same-day surgical unit of University Hospital, watching blood drip from a bag of whole blood attached to an infusion pole. And as Dr. Sparrow had explained, the nurses were quite thorough and ensured I was given the blood most compatible with mine. But I was reminded of once seeing lightening strike the same tree twice. (Why do we always seem to remember things that can add to our anxiety when facing a life challenge?)

As I lay on the hospital bed receiving the blood (it's like being low on iron and eating a big hunk of liver. The energy boost is incredible, if you can stand the taste of liver), I thought of the person from whom the blood came. I had no idea of the gender or race of the donor. I didn't know whether it was from a Democrat, Independent, or Republican, or if the person was vegetarian or a meat eater. I had no animosity or bias. I didn't care. I was only grateful that someone was thoughtful enough to make a donation. The situation further emphasized my belief that our souls are from the same entity—there is only one God—and He lives within each one of us. It is only physical appearance and language that separate us, both of which often promote hatred that leads to wars and destruction throughout the world.

Was I afraid of this operation? Yes, but only of the unknown. Dr. Sparrow had explained the procedure and I felt confident that he would do everything within his power to remove all of the cancer. Could I endure it? Absolutely. With Debbie's input, I knew I wanted to continue my war on cancer with every ounce of my focus. I wanted to live and enjoy the beauty of this earth. There were a lot of good years left in me, and I wanted to share them with the woman I loved.

Was it worth it? Definitely. And if confronted with the same choices, I'd opt for an instant replay.

Eight hours after the transfusion had begun, I walked to my car feeling better than I had in six months. The transfusion was already working, and it tasted much better than eating a slab of liver smothered in onions, bacon, and apples. I had a renewed source of power, even if it was temporary. No matter what future awaited me, I was going to enjoy every breath I took for the next week.

CHAPTER 3

Operation and Recovery

I ARRIVED at University Hospital at five thirty on Thursday morning with Debbie and her mother, Donna, who had arrived from Wisconsin a few days earlier to offer support. My mother, a lifetime smoker, had died thirty years before from lung cancer at age fifty-five, and so Donna's presence meant a great deal to me.

I kissed and hugged them both in the waiting room. Then I was escorted down a long corridor by a surgical nurse. I was optimistic, had confidence in my surgeon, and was eager to get through this part of the battle. Though I kept a smile on my face as I left Debbie, I was as frightened as I had been the day I first arrived in Vietnam. It was a lonely, gut-wrenching feeling. Anxiety coursed through me and I wasn't ashamed to admit it. As soon as I was hooked to an IV, the drugs began flowing, and the last thing I remember was telling Dr. Sparrow and Dr. Stone (who had agreed to assist) to tell my wife I loved her and to "Get it all."

I remember nothing about the operation, nothing about the recovery room, and I have only a vague memory of the two days following the operation. I felt little or no pain due to the morphine I received intravenously. The machine was hooked to an IV pole and was programmed with pre-measured doses I self-administered whenever I wanted; not a good idea. In a very short time I was as much an addict as someone who had been shooting up for years.

I've always viewed drug use as a way to escape reality and avoid responsibility, especially after witnessing the rebellion of the 1960s and 70s. But the 60s and 70s were innocent compared to the amount of drugs consumed by our troops in Vietnam. I've always liked being in control, but with morphine running through my veins, I felt numb and had little power over my senses;

something that has always been important in my life. I realized that drugs were helping me with the pain, but I also knew that drugs could be as deadly as the cancer that had been removed from my colon.

Vietnam caused more pain and suffering than I imagined possible. The physical pain began when I returned from war and realized I had malignant melanoma, but I lived daily in Vietnam with the emotional pain of being away from those I loved, and the spiritual pain of taking a human life.

We were all soldiers doing what we believed was right to keep America free. We all had families waiting for our safe return to the United States, but the pressure, horror, and loneliness of war is like a rapidly growing cancer—the effects were different for each soldier. Opium, heroin, and marijuana were frequent choices for solace and companionship. But drugs were temporary, and the reality of loneliness always returned. Some became addicted and some overdosed and died. A few went on shooting rampages and disappeared in the jungle, never to be seen again. But there is a story that I found more tragic than any other, one that could have become a nightmare for any of us who served in Vietnam, a story that has been repeated in every war.

I knew him as Michael. He was more of an acquaintance than a friend, but we sometimes talked when together in groups. He was a twenty-four-year-old Irishman, married to his high school sweetheart. He had a two-year-old son. He was short, stocky, and powerful—his thickness is most likely what kept him from being a "tunnel rat" (soldiers who performed underground search-and-destroy missions through tunnels created by the Viet Cong during the Vietnam War)—with no neck and a handshake like a vise. And this guy was incredibly funny. On more than one occasion, he sprayed shaving cream in the hand of a sleeping officer and then tickled the officer's nose with a feather. You can imagine what happened. And with a wee bit of an accent, his Irish jokes ignited laughter from everyone.

Michael loved to drink beer and fight, and he was good at both. He could drink a case of Budweiser in a couple of hours, which usually provoked his quick temper and nearly always led to a fight, which he usually won. But I later learned his preferred choice of companions was opium—his real escape from the war each night after the beer and fight.

He had been in-country for seven months when the world as he knew it crashed: a "Dear John" letter came from his wife. He was tormented day and night. The beer and fights increased, as did the opium. Finally, he snapped. I wasn't there when it happened, but I heard stories from a host of witnesses.

It was one in the morning when Michael took a .45 and a handful of loaded clips and sat down in the middle of the compound, his back against a sandbag bunker. He was stoned and dressed only in his boxers. Firing aimlessly into the dark sky, he captured the attention of nearly the entire compound in a few minutes.

He kept everyone frozen by threatening to kill anyone who came close. "It doesn't matter to me," he was quoted. "I'm done here and I'll take out anyone who tries to stop me." Each time he fired into the night he yelled, "Bitch!" When he exhausted a magazine, he quickly reloaded. Two MPs arrived and aimed their M-16s at his chest. They ordered him to surrender.

Michael again fired into the night and yelled, "Bitch!"

Both MPs fired rounds into the sandbags about five feet above Michael's head. Michael sat straight. His pained expression turned to laughter as if the monster had consumed him. Suddenly he began sobbing uncontrollably like a frightened child, and, with trembling hands, he put the gun to his temple and pulled the trigger.

The pressure, horror, and loneliness of war can be a hell on earth to many. In some ways, it's the same as the pain and suffering from inoperable cancer. Michael was another casualty of war, not a hero who died while saving his fellow soldiers, but one who died from his own internal suffering. Although he still had a son— an incredible reason to fight and return home— he simply lost the will to live.

I've never liked taking drugs of any kind. Being high on life has always been good enough for me. Was I afraid and lonely in Vietnam? Yes, more so than I like to admit, but I refused to take anything illegal. Does it make me a better person than Michael or my Vietnam buddies? Does it make me less susceptible to cancer? No. It simply means that I made a different choice. By not giving in and joining the drugs, I believe I helped my spirit grow. Something happened when I heard Michael's story, something that touched me deep within. I was no different from Michael, and I knew the same thing could have happened to me. It was my first real lesson as to how vulnerable we all are to the pain and suffering of life challenges. It's only our choices that separate us.

Michael gave up. But in my physical and emotional fight against cancer, I would not. As I said earlier, "Never…ever…give up! Never!"

Though I was riding an eight-mile-high morphine-induced cloud during my first days of recovery at University Hospital, there are several hallucinations that were more vivid than reality that I still remember with preciseness. *The Night Shift Urinal Conspiracy* was one of those hallucinations, and another reason why taking too many drugs can be dangerous.

At some point during my morphine-induced coma, the catheter inserted during the operation had been removed. Just before midnight—on the second day after surgery—I could not locate the urinal that I assumed would be hanging on the bed rail. I groggily searched the room, but it was nowhere to be found. However, luck was on my side and I spotted it hanging on the wall opposite the foot of the bed. It was painted with blue and white flowers that matched the wallpaper. Sabotage and conspiracy were written all over this. But I wasn't one to be fooled easily—they certainly weren't going to outwit me.

I maneuvered the sheet down to my knees, raised the hospital gown, took aim, and let loose a geyser that soaked the bottom half of the bed. I had them where I wanted them. But in the middle of feeling great satisfaction, a nurse, most likely the ringleader, walked in and yelled for help. This part I remember clearly, but what happened next is Debbie's narration.

I yelled at everyone in the room the entire time they were changing my sheets, unveiling their devious plot to hide the urinal. The shift supervisor ("Wendy" was on her name badge) quickly got Debbie on the phone. Twenty minutes later Debbie was standing by me holding my hand. I wasn't told whether I was given a sedative, but she held my hand and stayed by my side until I was asleep.

I woke again at one in the morning when a nurse checked my IV. I was immediately suspicious. She reminded me of one of the mama-sans who did my laundry in Vietnam. Was she slipping me truth serum to make me talk? No matter what torture awaited me, I would only give my name, rank, and serial number. Or, God forbid, was she giving me death juice? I remained cool and pretended to sleep, yet I kept one eye slightly open so I could follow every move she made. After she left, my anger grew—I spotted the camouflaged urinal still hanging on the wall. I didn't have to urinate, but it was the humiliation of being in the middle of a conspiracy and the fact that the nurse might have already injected embalming fluid into my IV that led to my next move. I had to be quick. If I was going out, I wasn't going quietly. So I ripped the IV out of my forearm and yelled like Rambo on the attack.

Within seconds blood covered my arm, gown, and the freshly changed sheets. The same nurse reentered the room and yelled for help. Again, there was momentary bedlam as all the conspirators helped change the sheets and start a new IV. As you may have already guessed, the cowards, most likely wanting to get me court-martialed, again called Debbie. She was by my side in twenty minutes, after having just fallen asleep at home. Needless to say, she was not at all pleased with my behavior, but she calmed me and again I floated away into oblivion. The head nurse ordered her to stay, and so each night until my discharge, either she or our daughter, Amanda, who was twenty and a full-time student at Santa Domingo College, slept curled like a cat in a chair until the enemy granted us a rollout bed. One of them had to be with me at all times.

It was the second incident that night that finally exploded common sense like fireworks through the warped minds of the enemy: take him off the morphine. And so my recovery began.

The following morning I was moved to a private room. Without morphine-saturated cells in my body, I was hurting.

"On a scale of one to ten, how is your pain?" the nurse asked, entering the room after

I had nearly destroyed the call button. Sandy was her name, and she was middle-aged and plump with short brown hair parted like a man's. What I remember most about her, other than her great bedside manner, is that she had the longest black eyelashes I had ever seen. Debbie later told me they were fake, but I didn't care—I thought they were beautiful.

I looked at the smiley-face chart for pain, which was attached to the wall in every patient's room, although some faces weren't so smiley. The first face had a zero underneath it and a happy, pain-free, Jimmy Carter smile. As the number under each face increased, indicating the severity of the patient's pain, the face gradually lost its smile until the number-ten face indicated the patient was in horrific pain beyond human comprehension. The face was frightening and reminded me of how I must have looked when I had previously suffered from a kidney stone.

"I don't really know how to answer that," I said, in obvious pain. It was difficult to relate to one of the smiley faces, but it certainly wasn't one of the first five.

"I'm not supposed to tell you this," Sandy said, "but your pain must be at the number six level or greater before I can give you any medication."

"It's at least a seven," I replied without hesitation, "or maybe an eight." Later I learned, whether it was true or not, to use the number eight when asking for meds.

She gave me Percoset, no morphine, and after twenty minutes of easier breathing, Sandy returned and changed the bandage covering the incision from the operation. It was the first time I had taken a look; a stapled ten-inch scar that began three inches above my navel took a direct southerly course through the navel, which baffled me (couldn't they have moved the incision at least a half inch in either direction), and ended at the beginning of where my pubic hair used to be.

The reality of what I had been through hit me like a slap in the face. I felt nauseous as Sandy cleaned the wound. The soft pressure of her fingers sent ripples of pain through my abdomen, but I drifted away to Roatan, Honduras, to the turquoise bay just down the road from a house Debbie and I had rented several years ago. It was a place I often went to in my mind as an escape from the trials and tribulations of life and, of course, pain. It worked until Sandy had finished cleaning the wound and applying a new bandage, and then I returned.

Debbie had been in the cafeteria for a cup of coffee and walked in just as I announced I had to relieve myself. I waited for Sandy to help me with the urinal, which was now a translucent plastic jug hooked on the side of the bed and no longer camouflaged in the wallpaper, but instead she moved it farther away from me.

"You need to pee, then use the toilet in the bathroom," she said.

My jaw must have dropped two feet. "I can hardly move," I complained. "Just give me the urinal." But she had now made it a game by sliding the jug to the end of the rail.

Debbie was doing everything she could to keep a straight face.

Sandy said again, "You want to pee, get out of the bed." She paused and gave me a watered down version of "the look." "And there had better be no accidents."

Maybe I had been wrong about Sandy. Maybe she was part of a new conspiracy. I wasn't very happy, but with Sandy and Debbie's help I shuffle-stepped to the bathroom. It took almost eight minutes to travel twenty feet, but it only took five minutes to return to the bed. I was exhausted, but I had literally taken the first steps to recovery.

By the end of the day I had graduated to unaccompanied bathroom trips while pushing the portable IV still hooked to my forearm. Regardless of the pain, I was unstoppable. It felt great to be out of bed and somewhat in control. Just before I retired for the night, and, of course, with Debbie's help—she was still required to remain overnight with me, just in case—I walked out of my room, hunched and still shuffle-stepping, and made it to the nurses' station. It felt as if I had just run a marathon, and my reward was a ride back to my room in a wheelchair.

"No pain medication," I told Wendy, the petite middle-aged blonde nurse who had reinserted my IV the night before after I had yanked it out of my arm. But after an hour of uninterrupted pain, I changed my mind.

Wendy was proud of me. "Don't be a hero," she warned. "If you really need the meds, take them." She also told me that I had only been one incident away from being transferred to the top floor of the hospital, the floor with padded walls and straitjackets and tranquilizers. For avoiding that, I knew I had Debbie to thank.

"Thanks," I said to Wendy. "I'm sorry for what I did last night. I know your job is tough enough without a problem patient."

She gave me an enormous smile, one that would have warmed the heart of Cinderella's evil stepmother.

Growing up, my father crammed being a man down my throat: no crying, be tougher than others, and never show your true feelings. My mother, however, told me on more than one occasion that it was easier to catch bees with honey than vinegar—such an easy concept yet so hard to implement. But can you really be a man and still show love, kindness, and compassion to others? Absolutely. Try it—you'll see how it makes you even more of a man. My advice when dealing with doctors and nurses and others in the medical profession is not to treat them as gods, but treat them with the same kindness and respect that you want them to show you. Kindness begets kindness; smiles beget smiles. But just as easily, rudeness begets rudeness and constant complaining begets strife.

Early the next morning I saw Dr. Sparrow. He was pleased with the progress I had made and upgraded my diet from liquid to soft, which made me extremely happy. Now that I was coherent, he explained that he had removed about a foot of my colon and that the adjacent lymph nodes showed no sign of cancer. "Everything looks good," he said.

This was the first information about the surgery we had heard, other than Dr. Sparrow informing Debbie immediately after the surgery that it had gone much as he had expected. It was great news, and I thought that I was not only on my way to a great recovery, but that I was rid of the cancer once and for all.

By the end of the day I was still on a natural high, had no IV, and was walking a marathon around the entire fifth floor. It was a great day—until I was summoned by the bathroom god. Ten minutes on the porcelain throne and my smiley face number was approaching eight. The blame was all mine, as I had coaxed an extra portion of soft food from one of the nurses—another bad idea. I should have left the healing to nature, but as often is the case, I was anxious, or stubborn, and tried to expedite the process. My advice is to be patient and not to overeat no matter how delicious a hospital soft diet looks.

My fourth and fifth days in the hospital were uneventful. I gained strength by the hour, and though I was still slightly hunched, my steps were no longer shuffles. My diet was still soft and the porcelain throne was now my friend.

My sixth and final day was greatly anticipated. After breakfast a student nurse, with my approval and under the direction of Nurse Sandy, clipped and removed the staples binding my incision. When she had finished, she beamed with pride. I was more than happy to contribute to the education of a future nurse. I knew she was going to be a good one.

By noon I was checked out of the hospital and waiting for my chariot when a woman I had never seen before entered the room. Tall, thin, and dressed in a navy pinstriped suit, she was in her mid-to-late forties with jaw-length black hair streaked with several thin strips of white. She reminded me a little of Cruella De Vil. "Hello, Mr. Yates," she said professionally without a smile as she extended her hand, "I'm Dr. Rosen, your oncologist."

The surprise on my face was evident, and I felt my jaw drop several inches, but it appeared to have little effect on Dr. Rosen. "I don't have an oncologist," I said frankly, the sting of her words sent a rush of bile to my throat.

Debbie stepped forward and introduced herself.

"Maybe we should sit for a moment," said Dr. Rosen.

Debbie and I sat on the side of the hospital bed while Dr. Rosen pulled up a chair and sat facing us. "This is just a preliminary meeting," she said. "I should have been here yesterday, but my schedule has been extremely hectic."

"And this is about chemotherapy?" I asked.

"Yes. Dr. Sparrow said he has already discussed this with you."

"We discussed the possibility." I paused. "As far as I know there was no final decision."

"I've talked with Dr. Sparrow and read your file. We both agree that chemotherapy will give you the best chance for a full recovery."

I was stunned. Bile was already burning my throat. The physical and emotional cliff I had worked so hard to climb over the past several days now seemed like wasted effort. I felt as if I were in a storm and the angry ocean had roared over the sides and into my boat. I've heard dozens of horror stories from friends and/or friends of friends who were sentenced to chemotherapy; some recovered, some died, and many of those who did survive were never the same, enduring fatigue, nausea, and cognitive impairment such as memory loss, forgetfulness, and extreme agitation.

Debbie sensed my anguish and asked, "Why do you think he needs chemotherapy?"

Dr. Rosen cocked her head and said matter-of-factly, "Do you want him to die?"

Debbie and I glanced at each other, each feeling pain from the slap of her words. We were too stunned to speak, so we shook our heads.

"I wouldn't be here if he didn't need chemotherapy," she said. She explained that although Dr. Sparrow had done a fine job with the surgery, the cancer had broken through my colon and was considered stage 2-B, which meant the tumor had the potential to extend to adjacent tissue or organs. She spent a full thirty minutes explaining the stages of colon cancer and her recommendations for follow-up treatments. "However, although I strongly recommend that you follow my advice, the decision is ultimately yours."

As I listened, the enthusiasm I felt about leaving the hospital was overtaken by anxiety and uncertainty. What was I going to do? I certainly didn't want to die. But what if the cure was worse than the disease? There was no way I could make such an involved decision at the moment.

Dr. Rosen left just as the wheelchair arrived for my voyage home. By now it was clear that this was not going to be a pleasure cruise. I had learned from Dr. Sparrow and the nurses that the next two weeks of recuperation were going to be physically taxing, yet I was confident I could handle it just as I had managed other recoveries. But chemotherapy? It was such an unknown at the time that I was reluctant to even consider it. My gut reaction was that there was no way I was going through chemotherapy, but according to Dr. Rosen it was something that needed to be done to increase the chance of a full recovery, and it was a decision I was going to have to make soon.

What I didn't know was that the demands of physical recovery over the next couple of weeks would be like a stroll on a Maui beach compared to the physical and emotional demands of chemotherapy.

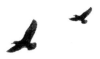

CHAPTER 4

Five Stages of Colon Cancer

DR. ROSEN explained that, as with each form of cancer, there are different stages of growth at the time of the tumor's discovery. The medical community recognizes five stages of colon cancer: stage 0, stage 1, stage 2-A and 2-B, stage 3, and stage 4. With each of these stages, with the sometimes exception of stage 4, the initial treatment is surgery to remove the diseased portion of the colon.

Stage 0

At this stage, the tumor is confined to the innermost lining of the colon, the mucosa, but regardless of the 0 rating, it is still considered cancer. A normal procedure for treatment is a colonoscopy or polypectomy, a local incision to remove the polyp and a small area of the tissue surrounding it. However, depending on the size of the tumor, more invasive surgery may be required to remove the diseased portion of the colon and reconnect the healthy tissue to sustain normal bowel function. Most physicians agree that the results of these procedures are considered curative and chemotherapy is not needed at this stage.

Stage 1

In this stage, the tumor has spread beyond the mucosa to the second and/or third layers of tissue, the submucosa and muscularis externa, and could possibly be in the beginning stage of involving the inside wall of the colon, or serosa, but, at this point, it has not broken through the outer wall to surrounding tissue.

Treatment at this stage is surgery to remove the diseased portion of the colon as well as additional tissue adjacent to the tumor. As long as the additional tissue tests are negative, further treatment and/or chemotherapy are typically not needed.

Most oncologists concur that the five-year survival rate for stage 1, sometimes referred to as Dukes A colon cancer, is roughly 90–95 percent, plus or minus 2–3 percent.

Stage 2

This stage of colon cancer, sometimes called Dukes B, actually resembles stage 1 and is confirmed only by surgical removal of the tumor. It is stage 2 if the tumor has penetrated the external wall of the colon and/or entered into the abdominal cavity. This stage can further be divided into two stages of its own: stage 2-A and stage 2-B, which is confirmed only after surgery.

Stage 2-A cancer affects the exterior wall of the colon, the serosa, but is still limited to the colon and does not involve the abdominal cavity. Stage 2-B has grown through the serosa and affected surrounding tissue and possibly organs. However, in both stages 2-A and 2-B, there are no tumor cells found in adjacent lymph nodes and no distant metastasis.

Surgery at this stage is critical, but once the tumor has broken through the serosa and has potentially exposed the surrounding tissue, surgery is usually not enough. Without additional treatment, and depending on stage 2-A or 2-B, there can be as much as a 50 percent chance for reoccurrence of the cancer.

Dr. Rosen explained that, even with surgery, small numbers of the tumor cells had spread outside my colon and were not removed by the surgery. In fact, the surgery itself can help to spread these undetected cells into the surrounding tissue. These renegade cells constitute micrometastases and are the causes of reoccurrence of the disease after surgery. (She used a tube of glitter as an example. She explained that when the tube was sealed, the cancer was intact, but if the lid was off and the glitter spilled, the tiny particles were easily scattered. Finding every spec of glitter with the human eye was literally impossible.) This is the reason she was so adamant at the hospital about chemotherapy. "Without chemotherapy," she warned, "the chance of tumor reoccurrence in your situation is roughly 50 percent, which usually affects the liver and/or lungs. With chemotherapy, we can reduce that chance more than half, improving the five-year recovery rate to approximately 80 percent."

Stage 3

This stage of colon cancer is similar to stage 2-B in that the tumor has broken through the serosa and affected the surrounding tissue, but it has spread to one, two, or three lymph nodes (nodes throughout the body that produce and store cells that fight infection).

As with stage 2, surgery is necessary to remove the tumor and surrounding tissue, as well as the affected lymph nodes. Chemotherapy is not an option but a necessity if the individual wants to survive the disease. Radiation is also a choice if the tumor is large and invading the tissue surrounding the colon. This stage of colon cancer is often referred to as Dukes C.

With surgery and chemotherapy, an accepted five-year survival rate is roughly 60 percent, plus or minus 2–3 percent.

Stage 4

At this stage of the disease, sometimes called Dukes D, the cancer has spread outside the colon to other parts of the body, typically the liver and/or lungs, but can also include the pancreas, small intestine, or other pelvic organs.

Treatment for this stage includes surgery (if possible) of the diseased portion of the colon, as well as lymph nodes and parts of affected organs where the tumor may have spread. However, if the cancer is determined inoperable, chemotherapy and/or radiation are generally used as the only hope for survival, oftentimes only to relieve symptoms. The accepted rate for five-year survival, even with chemotherapy and/or radiation, is now reduced to 5–8 percent.

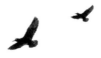

CHAPTER 5

Blockage

WALKING THROUGH the front door of my house was like reuniting with an old friend I hadn't seen in years. I wanted to bend down and kiss the floor as I had the ground when I first stepped off the chartered plane and onto U.S. soil after returning from Vietnam—but I couldn't bend at the waist. I said earlier that I didn't associate any of my battles with cancer with dying, but when I left the house early on the morning of the surgery, I had no idea how saturated my colon was with cancer, and I really didn't know if I would ever see home again.

I continued on the soft diet that Dr. Sparrow prescribed for my first two weeks at home. It consisted mostly of liquids, Jell-O, protein drinks, soup, yogurt, and chocolate and tapioca pudding. There wasn't much else I could handle the first few days, but it mattered little because my appetite was minimal—I had already lost twenty pounds.

I walked twice a day, morning and evening, each a marathon that bested my previous record, and after five days, I was walking fully erect for approximately a mile a day. Was it difficult? Yes, but having enjoyed physical activity all of my life gave me incentive to push myself.

Debbie had returned to work for a few days but called often to check on me. My appetite had suddenly increased and I was now devouring everything soft I could find; my personal favorite was two eggs over easy smothering instant grits.

I had been home a full week and I felt great. I was off all pain medication, physically improving every day, and maintaining my soft diet. When I woke on Tuesday morning I felt stronger than ever after a sound sleep. I was starving, so I joined Debbie and her mother in the kitchen. They were very excited to see me so chipper and ready for a great day. Debbie had taken the day off to take her mother to the airport. They were just finishing breakfast at the kitchenette as I began cooking eggs to accompany my instant grits, but I was famished and wanted something more substantial. Since the toaster was already out, I decided on a sourdough English muffin coated with a healthy layer of crunchy peanut butter and Wisconsin cherry jam. My diet was supposed to be completely soft for another week, but after all, I was healing ahead of schedule. A muffin with crunchy peanut butter and jam sounded delicious and should be no problem, right? Another of my dumb ideas.

By eleven o'clock, my severe abdominal pain equaled at least a number seven smiley face on the pain chart. Nauseous, I eased into bed after swallowing two Vicodin.

Debbie was only minutes from taking her mother to LAX for a three thirty departure. Instead, she phoned the local shuttle company and found a bus leaving in half an hour. "Don't move!" she fired at me as she and her mother loaded the car. There was no need for her to worry. I knew that if I moved I would lose everything in my stomach, which maybe wasn't such a bad idea, although it would probably rip open my incision.

She returned in twenty-five minutes and placed a call to Dr. Sparrow. He was in surgery at University Hospital, so his nurse advised her to get me to the emergency room as quickly as possible. My smiley-face pain was an eight as I hobbled to the car, and Debbie, who has always thought she was born to be a NASCAR driver, had us at the emergency room in ten minutes. But, just like the military, it was hurry up and wait.

The emergency room was standing room only: mothers with crying babies, screaming kids with cuts and broken bones, and those with coughs and runny noses were abundant. After one couple was called by a nurse, Debbie and I found seats at the rear of the waiting room next to a make-shift play station for kids. I waited through twenty minutes of mind-boggling pain, twisting and tucking and desperately seeking a comfortable position that would at least take me back to a six or seven smiley face before seeing the intake nurse. When my time finally arrived, the nurse was sympathetic to the amount of pain I was experiencing and immediately sent us to the same-day surgical area that was used as a backup when the number of emergencies was heavy.

There were two potential patients with family members already sitting in a row of folding chairs lining the wall when we arrived. Several minutes elapsed before a nurse came into the hallway and asked each of us the nature of our complaint. One patient was a large middle-aged man with a nasty cough that resembled chain-smoker hacking, the other was an elderly woman who hiccupped every ten to twenty seconds and appeared exhausted and fragile from two days of continuous hiccupping. To my surprise, when Debbie explained my problem, the nurse took me right away.

Her name was Rachael, and, believe it or not, she was even kinder and more compassionate than Sandy, the nurse I had grown so fond of during my hospital stay. She was in her late thirties with shoulder-length curly hair the color of chestnuts, a smile full of dimples, and a deep concern and dedication for those she helped. She was truly a credit to her profession.

Debbie relayed a short version of the past two weeks and Rachael immediately started an IV. Twenty minutes later Dr. Sparrow entered the room and ordered pain medication, and within seconds, my smiley-face number dropped to two.

By now it was one in the afternoon and what I heard, I didn't like. "There appears to be some form of blockage," I heard Dr. Sparrow tell Debbie, though his words seemed broken and somewhat slow. "Is he still on the soft diet I prescribed?"

Debbie explained what I had eaten for breakfast. "What do we do now?" she asked.

"The first thing we do is pump his stomach, and then we find the cause."

By now I was riding a magic carpet and feeling no pain, but I was still lucid enough to understand every word. "I'm not getting my stomach pumped," I argued, but it also sounded as though my own words were in slow motion, and no one was listening. "Let's just wait for it to pass."

My words fell on deaf ears because Rachael forced me into a wheelchair and rolled me, as fast as NASCAR Debbie drove to the hospital, to a cubicle in the emergency room. Within minutes, she had inserted a tube up my right nostril and into my stomach. I gagged and vomited twice. Debbie cried and left the room.

Rachael was satisfied with the insert and hooked the tube to a pump. Within seconds a circular container attached to the pump filled with a green solution that looked and smelled like rancid pea soup. It was enough to make everyone who looked at it gag, but my nausea instantly subsided.

I remained in the cubicle until the tube insertion and pump were checked by the emergency room physician and everyone was satisfied that I was stable, and then I was moved to a semi-private room. I was no longer nauseous, so, of course, I wanted a tray of the same food the guy next to me had just received. Not a chance.

Debbie didn't have to remain overnight with me because I wasn't on morphine or hallucinating. The tube up my nose and into my stomach was foreign, but, with Ativan, I was handling it okay.

The following morning I underwent a series of X-rays after drinking a Barium solution the technician said "tastes like a strawberry milkshake." It was definitely nothing like a milkshake and tasted more like strawberry flavored chalk mixed with Play-Doh. I badgered the pimply-faced X-ray tech for any information pertaining to the blockage, but all he gave me were a few low grunts.

Debbie was in the room when I returned and spent the day with me awaiting word from Dr. Sparrow, but none came. I was famished, but until there was some explanation for what had caused me pain and whether or not there was a blockage (which could mean another surgery), I was sentenced to starvation.

Dr. Sparrow finally entered the room at five thirty. "How would you like that removed?" he asked, pointing to the tube in my nose.

A smile lit my face as if I had just won the lottery. I wanted to kiss him. I was so emotional that all I could do was nod.

I thought it might be as difficult to get it out as it was putting it in, gagging and vomiting and Debbie crying as she ran from the room. I didn't care if I gagged and vomited (although I hated to see Debbie cry) as long as the plastic snake was removed, but to my surprise, Dr.

Sparrow reached up, grabbed the tube, and yanked it out. I sucked in a long breath, as if I had been holding my breath while underwater and had just reached the surface. It was one of the greatest feelings I've ever experienced.

"Okay," said Dr. Sparrow, "we found no blockage so you're good to go."

One thing I can tell you about Debbie is that since I've known her she has not and never will accept, "We found no blockage so you're good to go," and just leave it at that. Unlike me, she wants to know everything about everything: the way it works, why it works, the way it smells, the sequence of events, what's going to happen next, and why it happened. I was grateful that the tube was out, and Dr. Sparrow's words were enough for me, but I was elated that she cared enough about me to want to know more. And any information could help prevent a similar situation in the future.

"What was the problem?" she asked.

"One of several things," said the doctor. "It could be the scar tissue already building in the area of reattachment, and the colon is still somewhat swollen, or it could also be the bread and crunchy peanut butter."

Debbie cut her eyes at me before looking at Dr. Sparrow. "Is there a chance that this could happen again?"

"Yes."

I knew at this point I needed to join the conversation. "Then how long should I continue on the soft diet?"

"For at least the next week," Dr. Sparrow replied. "The swelling should subside by that time. But when you do begin to eat solid food, introduce it gradually and in moderation."

"And then he doesn't have to worry about what he eats?" Debbie asked.

"I wish it was that easy," replied Dr. Sparrow, "but, unfortunately, it could happen again at any time—a week, a month, or even longer." A silent moment passed before he continued. "You want to get out of here?"

I smiled. "Absolutely."

Several hours later I was home and again eating soft food, but it wasn't the last blockage. I followed Dr. Sparrow's diet advice for another ten days just to make sure, but then I relented. I knew I didn't want to live the rest of my life without actually chewing food, and I didn't want to be so overcautious that I constantly worried about it, so that night I ate two slices of thick-crust vegetarian pizza.

Within two hours there appeared to be another blockage. I refused to go to the emergency room; I knew that if the toast and peanut butter had dislodged and eventually passed through the battle zone of my colon, chances were the pizza would do the same thing, at least I hoped it would. (I'm not advising anyone who faces a blockage after surgery to take matters into their own hands and follow the route I took. Instead, I recommend that you follow your doctor's advice, and if you think you might have a blockage, get to the emergency room as quickly as possible.) But knowing my own body and having just gone through a terrifying experience that I didn't want to repeat, I was hoping I could handle it myself, and frankly, I was both embarrassed and afraid to return to the ER. So I took two tablespoons of Milk of Magnesia and lay gingerly on the bed. Two hours of listening to my stomach gurgle resulted in no more pain or blockage, and then there was a hearty bowel movement. From observing the contents of the stool, I believe this blockage was due to undigested red bell peppers and the thick crust of the pizza. (Yes, that's just one of the skills you develop with colon cancer.)

A few days later I had yet another apparent blockage, this time from eating two Louisiana hot sausage dogs smothered in Dijon mustard and topped with grilled onions. Again I had severe pain and took the Milk of Magnesia and listened to my stomach gurgle for several hours, and then the blockage cleared. I think the difficulty this time was from the sausage casing, which my system had not digested. My suggestion is that once solid food is eaten, plenty of time should be taken to chew and grind the food well, extremely well. (Some nutritionists and physicians advise chewing each bite of a meal twenty-two times, which seemed to help me.)

A follow-up colonoscopy a year later indicated that the opening at the reattachment of my colon was healed, clear, and large enough to process food. Though it's been over four years from the last blockage, the memory of the pain is a clear reminder of what could still happen. So knowing my own body and what it can process, I chose to eliminate certain foods from my diet. I still obsessively chew my food until it turns to mush, which means that I'm usually the last one to finish eating dinner each night. Each of us knows what is good for us and what is not if we listen to our bodies. By simply paying attention, we will understand what we should and should never eat.

I had survived the surgery, the hallucinations from morphine, and three blockages in my colon. I was getting stronger by the day and had gained a few pounds. Life was good again and I was sure that what I had gone through was well worth the pain, until I got the phone call from the one I had already labeled The Wicked Witch of the West—Dr. Rosen.

CHAPTER 6

Portacath

DR. ROSEN'S office was on the second floor of a seven-story medical office building adjacent to University Hospital. The medical center represented a wide variety of specialties in the medical profession: oncology, gastro-intestinal, X-ray, podiatry, infectious disease, and same-day surgery. There was also a well-equipped fitness center on the first floor for employees that equaled some of the leading private fitness clubs.

Debbie and I waited ten minutes before the lab tech took my blood pressure, weight, pricked my finger for a drop of blood, and then escorted us down a short hallway to a small examining room. Dr. Rosen entered ten minutes later. She wore a black skirt and white blouse, and with her black hair, which still had thin streaks of white, she looked more like Cruella De Vil than at the hospital. Pleasantries were exchanged, and then she said, "You're looking stronger."

"I'm feeling pretty good," I replied.

Debbie briefly explained the recent episodes with the blockage, but I could tell Dr. Rosen was listening cordially and really wanted to get down to the business in which she was an expert: chemotherapy.

"I think you're ready for this," she said.

I was still very apprehensive. "I don't know if I can do it."

Debbie cut her eyes at me, a gesture I had seen far too often over the past month. We had talked at great length as to why I should listen to the doctors. "I love you," she had said, "and I don't want to lose you. Chemotherapy can increase the odds that you will survive this."

Dr. Rosen had previously explained that there was perhaps a 50 percent chance that the cancer would return, and if it did, it would most likely affect my liver and/or lungs. But with chemotherapy, the percentage would be reduced to less than 25 percent, a number to which Debbie and I were much more receptive.

I stared hard at Dr. Rosen and realized my next question was one that Debbie normally asked. "I guess before I totally commit I need to know the game plan. Why do you think it will help me?"

"I believe in being extremely aggressive. In past years our best choice for success was using 5-Fluorouracil, or 5-FU, but we're now using it with Oxaliplatin with much greater success."

"Are you optimistic about my chances?" I asked.

"Mr. Yates," (she always referred to me this way), "I look at half a glass of water as half-full, not half-empty. With chemotherapy there are never any guarantees, but, in your case, with the chemotherapy treatment I prescribe, I would say that there is an excellent chance for a full recovery."

I liked her answers, especially about being aggressive. I suddenly saw her as Glinda the Good Witch. "Okay, I'll do it."

"Good," she replied with a smile. "I'll show you the treatment room in a few minutes, but first we need to discuss an IV port."

My first thought was the kind of IV port most commonly used, like the one that had been stuck in my forearm most of the last month and a half, but Dr. Rosen did not recommend this for longer periods of chemotherapy. "With one or two treatments," she said, "a normal IV port would probably work; although, there would still be a lot of sticks, but a longer treatment can collapse the veins and is not very practical."

Then she explained an Implantable Venous Access Port, sometimes called a Portacath, which is a reservoir (portal) of plastic, stainless steel, or titanium with a silicone bubble (septum) for needle insertion with an attached catheter. The half-moon and quarter-shaped device is surgically inserted under the skin, usually in the upper chest or arm and appears as a bump under the skin—imagine a one-inch-diameter jawbreaker cut in half with the crescent portion as the bump. During the surgery, a procedure performed under local anesthesia with aid-imaging guidance, usually X-ray or ultrasound, the catheter is inserted into a vein, ideally the right internal jugular, if possible. Because of the scars on the right side of my neck from the earlier melanoma surgeries, the catheter was inserted into my left internal jugular vein with the septum just above my left breast. This connection allows the chemotherapy to spread quickly and efficiently throughout the body—like an invading army of sword-swinging molecules searching for the enemy.

The septum is made of self-sealing silicone that resembles a tiny pin cushion. It can receive hundreds of punctures without damage and is ideal for long-term use.

"This is definitely the method to use," Dr. Rosen recommended. "It will be much easier for you and us."

"Who does this procedure?" Debbie asked.

"It's a surgical procedure, so I'll set it up with Dr. Sparrow."

I had gotten to know Dr. Sparrow quite well over the past month and I liked him, but I wasn't looking forward to seeing him again so soon. However, if I was going to have it done, I was glad he would do it.

Debbie and I were given a tour of the treatment room and introduced to the two oncology nurses, Michelle and Sherri. Michelle was in her early thirties, tall with the body of a distance runner, brown straight hair she usually kept in a ponytail, and a smile that complemented her trusting demeanor. Sherri, on the other hand, was the epitome of a disciplined military nurse. Short and slightly overweight, she had red curly hair and was probably around fifty. She always presented herself as the One in Charge. She reminded me of the old sergeant major at Fort Gordon almost thirty-five years ago—shrapnel sharp, rugged exterior, and a heart as big as a refrigerator.

The room was large and much cooler than the waiting and examining rooms. The air was permeated with an unfamiliar chemical smell. A fourth of the room was similar to a nurses' station where chemical cocktails were mixed, with a computer station to log them. The remainder of the room contained eight brown recliners set in a crescent-moon arrangement with an infusion pole and monitor beside each one.

Debbie and I sat on folding chairs off to the side observing the activity in the room. The nurses were pretty incredible. As I watched them taking care of six patients, I wondered why they had chosen their profession. I don't think it was for the money because I have never seen two people who displayed more kindness and compassion to those they we treating.

Once, during my chemotherapy treatments, Michelle was on vacation. Her replacement was a three on my one-to-ten rating scale for chemotherapy nurses. Maybe I was just used to the normal caring and kindness Michelle and Sherri brought with them every day they came to work. Maybe I was secretly in love with Michelle and would not have accepted anyone who tried to replace her. Whatever it was, I wasn't happy. The new nurse was professional at all times (I had observed Michelle and Sherri enough during the hooking and unhooking procedures to know what to expect), but for some reason, she wasn't a happy person to be around. And caring, kindness, and compassion seemed as though they were an afterthought and forced.

I sat for a long moment staring at an empty recliner picturing myself totally controlled by chemicals. It seemed so foreign, so surreal, yet I knew that soon enough I would be one of many in this world undergoing chemotherapy. I shared a common goal with the strangers in this room: we wanted to live.

I had a good primary care physician, a good surgeon, and I hoped I was going to be happy with my oncologist, but I was ecstatic about having Michelle and Sherri taking care of me. It certainly had a positive effect on my mental outlook heading into my first chemotherapy treatment. Chemotherapy is a trying time, so please be sure you are happy with those treating you. It is that important.

I was full of questions: What would happen to me? Would I lose my hair? Would the chemicals harm my body more than they would help? I didn't like the unknown and I really didn't want to undergo chemotherapy, yet I had survived the unknown day to day for a year in Vietnam and lived to tell about it. Could this be any worse?

Sitting in the treatment room, I had the first of many bouts with nausea from what many refer to as "chemo day." But as Debbie squeezed my hand, I was reminded of the reason I needed to accept this part of my life challenge.

Life challenges can be extremely difficult, and I can't imagine having to face this one alone. Have you ever loved someone so much that just being with them was worth all of the trials and tribulations of living on this earth, and the life challenges we must face? That's how it was and is with Debbie. And, oh, how I wanted to live. Am I lucky, or what? Good or bad, I had someone to stand beside me and would be in this with me to the end. I wasn't going to run away or hide my head in the sand. I had to fight it with every ounce of my total being. It was for Debbie, and it was for me.

The following Thursday, Dr. Sparrow performed the thirty-minute Portacath procedure under local anesthesia at University Hospital. The port implant was successful and I was in and out of the hospital in four hours. Was I frightened? Without a doubt. But as I explained earlier, it was only of the unknown. Ativan at the time of the IV hookup helped my anxiety. All in all, it was as easy as having the colonoscopy.

It might sound as though I take Ativan on a regular basis; not true. I do take a prescribed .5 milligram tablet when I know I'm going to be under stress: dentist and doctor visits and flying. Don't be afraid to talk to your doctor or anesthesiologist about easing your anxiety. They are actually more human and understanding than we perceive them to be. There is no need to suffer from stress-related situations.

Ten days of healing and another office visit with Dr. Sparrow and I was pronounced "good to go" for chemotherapy. It was not what I considered my lucky day.

The very next day, Friday, was my final appointment with Dr. Rosen before actually beginning chemotherapy. She was pleased that the port was satisfactorily in place and that I had certainly recovered from the surgery. "We shouldn't waste another moment," she said, and then scheduled my first treatment for Monday morning.

As Debbie and I left the medical center, I breathed deeply. Somehow, sucking in the fresh coastal air helped calm the nausea that threatened every time I was in Dr. Rosen's office or anywhere near the treatment center.

"Are you okay?" Debbie asked.

I sucked in another long breath. "Yes, but let's get out of here and do something fun. I don't want to think about Monday morning until I actually have to."

She took my hand in hers and smiled. "Later. We're off to another appointment."

CHAPTER 7

Magic Mushrooms

THE NEXT appointment was with a licensed nutritionist, Shannon LaBre, whom Debbie had known for many years. Actually, some nineteen years earlier I had also worked briefly with Shannon at a small health care group after I first moved to Southern California.

Shannon was in her early fifties, an eternal hippie, and one of those seemingly rare individuals whose smile exemplifies her love for life and engulfs everyone in complete acceptance. Her lion-mane hair was riddled with gray and she wore a colorful bag dress and sandals as she sat behind a small, cluttered desk. She was definitely a free spirit, yet she exuded professionalism that I knew came from her nutritional knowledge and understanding.

With Shannon, "What you see if definitely what you get."

We talked about nutrition, diets, and cancer for almost half an hour. Much of what she recommended I already knew from Internet medical and nutrition sites. I've always been fascinated with herbs and holistic medicine—at an earlier time in my life, I was heavily involved in health food stores, vitamins, natural foods, and sports— but Shannon really piqued my interest when she suggested a supplement to my diet, especially while I was undergoing chemotherapy: Coriolus VPS, a Japanese mushroom extract that I began referring to as "magic mushrooms." If you think these mushrooms are hallucinogenic, think again. They are simply supplements to any diet.

During our meeting with Shannon, she made it perfectly clear that if it was her husband in my place, she would insist that he take the supplement. So when I got home, I immediately searched the Internet for hours to find more on these magic mushrooms. There wasn't much information available, but there was enough for me to realize that they could be beneficial in beating cancer.

Magic mushrooms are not widely recognized in the Western world (especially by most physicians) as beneficial for treatment of any cancer or problems arising from such treatment, but in the Eastern world, they are often a way of life. Research in Japan alone has existed for more than twenty-five years and reports incredible success stories regarding the healing properties of these mushrooms. Shannon also provided several examples of healing benefits to two cancer patients she had worked with after surgery—both patients were survivors of colon cancer. One, in particular, had already lived seven years past his physician-determined expiration date and was expected to live for many more years.

The active ingredients in this species of mushroom, Coriolus versicolor, are protein-bound polysaccharides that have demonstrated significant immuno-modulating properties.

Do they work? Were Shannon's patients' survival due to magic mushrooms? It's certainly possible. And Shannon is definitely a believer.

Though I am not suggesting that anyone with cancer try this supplement, I believe it was one of the many pieces of the puzzle that helped with my ultimate survival. I still take them daily.

How do I know they helped with my survival?

There are times in all of our lives when we feel deeply within our hearts that something is right, that it just makes sense. Perhaps there is no logical or physical evidence, but it's there within us. It's like Debbie's love for me—she doesn't have to outwardly express it; I feel her love with my soul just as one feels the spiritual connectedness to whatever form of God they choose to worship. How do you explain it? There is no all encompassing answer. You just know.

In many Japanese studies, magic mushrooms have proved beneficial in nutritional support with radiotherapy, after curative surgery for colon cancer, and with chemotherapy. These studies found that the five-year survival rate of patients who received Coriolus polysaccharides were, in most cases, doubled—some more than tripled—as opposed to those who did not use the mushrooms.

Dr. Rosen gave me a 50 percent chance of surviving colon cancer for five years without chemotherapy, and about a 75 percent chance with chemotherapy. By my calculation, including magic mushrooms with my diet and supplements would give me somewhere between a 90 and 95 percent chance to be cancer free at the end of five years. Not only did Debbie and I like the numbers, it was an easy choice for us.

Debbie and I agreed that I should take the magic mushrooms, but we also agreed that before I added the supplement to my diet, I should discuss it with Dr. Rosen. I ordered the mushroom supplement online and received them the following week, a three- to four-month supply for approximately two hundred dollars.

Is the cost more than vitamins? Yes.

Is the cost covered by insurance? No.

But as I said, some things you just know you have to do.

Would I do it again? Absolutely. I'm still taking them.

With a better understanding of the direction I was heading, and the expectancy of perhaps living longer with the magic mushrooms, Debbie and I felt more relief than we had in months. We went out to dinner Friday and Saturday night and spent Sunday together at church, lunch, and a movie; more than anything, we wanted to keep my mind off Monday morning.

During the weekend, I felt I could breathe a little easier and I presented a tranquil demeanor. I had another unknown to face on Monday, which I was determined to handle with confidence, but deep inside, I had the feeling that I was in the eye of a storm.

CHAPTER 8

Chemotherapy 1

MONDAY MORNING September 18 was my personal D-Day. I arrived at the medical center at nine for my first treatment. Debbie was beginning her final five weeks before retirement and had several meetings to attend, so a good friend, John, volunteered to help me weather the storm. Debbie was scheduled to pick me up at one o'clock.

John is retired and about fifteen years older than I am. At the time I began chemotherapy I was fifty-eight, so that put him around seventy-three. At seventy-three, he was a Mexican marine who was heavily decorated for his service to our country in Korea and Vietnam and a helluva man, one to emulate. I hope I'm at least half as active when I'm his age.

It took twenty minutes for Michelle and Sherri to fix my three-hour Oxaliplatin cocktail and hook it to the port in my chest. They had also been instructed by Dr. Rosen to add Ativan to help me relax, and, to my surprise, the hookup was no more painful than a pin prick. It was something I had worried over incessantly, so I wished I could have read about it before my first experience. It could have saved me a lot of grief.

I remember lying back in the recliner, my body rigid, my hands squeezing my thighs. It was the same position I assumed when reclined in a dentist's chair. Michelle explained each step as she hooked me up. Just listening to her reassuring voice calm me, and then she said, "You're going to feel a little stick." I tightened more, but that's really all it was: a little stick. It was nothing worse than a B-12 shot.

All of my worrying was for nothing, but I wondered if the stick was the easy or hard part of chemotherapy. Even with the Ativan I was still anxious, but John was right there with me telling me war stories and keeping my mind off the monster I was afraid would suddenly appear. Finally, my eyelids felt as if they had tiny weights attached. John kept talking and I kept doing my best to listen.

Michelle must have realized I was about to pass out because I vaguely remember her telling John that if he would allow me a few minutes alone I would totally relax and slip into a sea of tranquility. He left to use the restroom and the next thing I remember was Debbie sitting in the same chair John had occupied, holding my hand. It was twelve-twenty-five, and I had been floating through Wonderland chasing white rabbits for over two and a half hours, not knowing if I had been snoring, drooling, or both. John had returned briefly to check on me. "You were really out of it," he told me the next day.

Twenty minutes later a beep from the monitor signaled the end of my treatment. Michelle unhooked the IV from my port, gave the port a quick saline flush, and inserted another IV that she hooked to a battery-powered pump the size of a walkie-talkie, which clipped to my belt. Every five seconds the pump shot the deadly chemical 5-Fluorouracil, or 5-FU, through a tube into the port. There was enough 5-FU in the pump pouch for two days of treatment, and I was scheduled to return on Wednesday at noon to have it removed.

Dr. Rosen's plan was twelve treatments, one every other week: three hours of Oxaliplatin cocktails in the treatment room, two days at home on the 5-FU pump, and then a meeting with her on Friday to analyze the treatment, the side effects, and where we would go and how we would proceed.

Debbie took the rest of the day off and drove me home. There was really no need for her to be there because as soon as I hit the couch I was out for the next three hours. The effects of the 5-FU must have been instant because when I awoke I was nauseous. I managed to down a cup of soup for dinner, but nothing else other than a few sips of Gatorade. I knew I needed nourishment, but I just couldn't eat. The smell and sight of food was as sickening to me as changing a toddler's dirty diaper.

I had a miserable first night with the pump—every five seconds I heard a *click-clunk*, a nauseating sound that kept me awake in anticipation of the next *click-clunk*. I would eventually learn to ignore this sound, but it heightened the nausea that had overcome me. At nine o'clock Tuesday morning I was so sick that I drove myself back to the treatment room and lobbied several twelve-hour nausea pills from Dr. Rosen and a prescription for the same. (I would recommend that you have nausea pills in hand before leaving the treatment room after your initial session of chemotherapy. All you have to do is ask.)

Did the pills help? I think so, but the pills only did so much.

For the first week of treatment the nausea and I became one. Oftentimes I would lose the pills to the porcelain god shortly after I took them, so sometimes they weren't all that helpful.

Other than nausea, fatigue, and the *click-clunk* of the pump, Tuesday night and Wednesday morning were uneventful. I arrived at the treatment room at noon on Wednesday and within five minutes the pump was unhooked. I was a free man—at least for eleven more days. I had made it through the first chemo session and felt like celebrating. On the way home I stopped at a bakery and bought an apple fritter, a treat I've always enjoyed. I had no idea why I had a craving for such unhealthy food, but I had had little nourishment since Monday. At the time, I didn't realize that apple fritters would become the staple of my diet over the next three months. However, I was still so nauseous that I wanted nothing more than to remain perfectly still.

I've talked to cancer and chemotherapy survivors over the years and, in nearly all of the cases, there was a specific food that made their recovery more manageable: apple fritters, jelly doughnuts, cheese, rice, cucumbers, granola with honey, and a number of other foods. I don't know if it's the same for every chemotherapy survivor, but I haven't had an apple fritter since my last chemotherapy treatment. I'm sure it's psychological, but the sight of an apple fritter now sends a wave of nausea through me. I also believe that it's the association with the entire cancer experience. However, the physical symptoms are very real.

I had an office visit with Dr. Rosen on Friday to discuss the first session, and by then I had already experienced other side effects. I was still somewhat nauseous, although not as severely, and food had lost most of its appeal. In fact, my taste buds appeared to be in shock and unable to distinguish tastes, except for the sweetness of apple fritters.

I could not drink or touch anything cold; to do so would cramp my cheeks instantly and cause my fingers to throb and turn red. Dr. Rosen said the nausea and weird feeling in my fingers were expected, but she had never had a complaint regarding cramping cheeks. (Though she'd never had a patient complain of cramping cheeks, it was my body experiencing the side effects, and I know my cheeks cramped because of the treatment.) There was also an odd taste—maybe it was my good cells exploding—that remained with me the first week of each treatment. I've heard others refer to it as a "metallic taste," and, for the lack of a better description, I'll call it the same.

I continued to improve over the weekend and into Monday. By Tuesday morning the nausea had totally subsided and my appetite had returned, although my taste buds were still on vacation. I was hungry, but I found that eating food without the expected and familiar flavor didn't quite seem worth the effort.

Debbie encouraged me and always ate with me. I knew I needed the nourishment, but I was already looking forward to my next apple fritter, something I could actually taste.

Dr. Rosen considered my first chemotherapy session successful and believed that I would definitely be able to handle all twelve sessions. I had no idea what to expect going into the first treatment, and I had not experienced anything similar in any of my previous life challenges, but it was definitely more frightening than any situation I encountered in Vietnam. If I had to pick one side effect during my first treatment that I disliked the most, it had to be nausea. I think most of us who have gone through chemotherapy learn to live with some of the side effects, but I would wager that nausea is at the top of many lists.

On Friday afternoon I received the magic mushrooms I had ordered. I was excited and immediately opened the box and the first jar, but Debbie reminded me that we had agreed to let Dr. Rosen know before I began taking the supplement.

After calling and speaking with her coordinator, Dr. Rosen called back thirty minutes later. I explained the visit to the nutritionist and her recommendation and the benefits of taking the supplement, but she wasn't as receptive as I had hoped. In fact, she was making the Wicked Witch of the West look pretty good.

"Mr. Yates," I was starting to dislike this title, "I don't want you taking anything other than your prescribed medications while you are undergoing chemotherapy."

I was completely dumbfounded. "But, why? It's only a nutritional supplement, just like vitamins. And you advised me to keep taking a daily multivitamin because it could actually help me feel better. And what if it could really help increase my chances for a complete recovery?"

There was a pause before she spoke, firmly. "We have no knowledge that this mushroom supplement works." And then she asked me, "And what if the mushrooms have an adverse effect and hinder the Oxaliplatin and 5-FU?" Another moment of silence. "Mr. Yates, I am your oncologist, and if I'm going to treat you, you must follow my instructions."

I felt as if I had just been scolded by my fourth-grade teacher for dabbing the end of a long ponytail—the blonde hair of the cute girl who sat at the desk in front of me and the one I was secretly in love with—into a jar of paste. And I felt guilty; perhaps the same as Peter felt when he denied Jesus for the third time. "Okay," I relented, "I'll do it your way."

"Very well," she said, "then I'll see you again on Monday."

I hung up and stared at Debbie who sat on the opposite side of the breakfast table. There was a painful moment of silence before she said, "I'm sorry. I know how much you were looking forward to this."

I nodded, still dazed by my conversation with Dr. Rosen. I was trying very hard to understand why the medical profession refused to accept or recommend any supplement that did not require a prescription and FDA approval. However, Debbie was quick to point out the power of pharmaceutical companies, which dictated the actions of many physicians.

I accepted Dr. Rosen's decision for the time being, yet something within me understood that the magic mushrooms not only worked but would soon become part of my life. As soon as chemotherapy ended, I planned to add them to my daily diet. Regardless, I had only two days until my next treatment, and I wasn't going to allow what I considered a minor setback to interfere with my mental well-being.

The Wicked Witch of the West, Cruella De Vil, or even the Wicked Stepmother was not going to stop me. I was going to enjoy my weekend as best I could because I had no control over what awaited me on Monday.

CHAPTER 9

Chemotherapy 2

ON MONDAY morning October 2, John picked me up at 8:40 and drove me to the medical center. Debbie could have resumed responsibility, but I think John was feeling a connection and wanted to do something that made a difference in his life and mine. I was not only grateful for his concern and friendship, but I was also fortunate to have his company.

We arrived at nine sharp and I went to the same recliner as during my first treatment. John pulled a folding chair next to me and proceeded to talk my ear off. Fifteen minutes later my Oxaliplatin cocktail was ready and Michelle flushed my port and hooked me up.

First came the Ativan and then the cocktail, and within minutes I felt myself again following the white rabbit into Wonderland.

This time John took the cue, as I had closed my eyes and hadn't heard a word he said for at least a minute. He left quietly, sat in the waiting room for half an hour, and then checked to see how I was doing before he left the building. He was quite the mother hen.

I slept for an hour before my eyes popped open. An elderly woman two chairs from me apparently couldn't handle her cocktail. She was as pale as chalk and was barfing into a round plastic bowl provided by Drill Sergeant Sherri. I, too, was feeling a touch of nausea from the sound, but I soon forgot about myself as I witnessed one of the most beautiful displays of human compassion I had ever seen. Vomit had splashed on Sherri's blouse and arms, but she was focused on calming the woman, changing the liner in the bowl, and dabbing the woman's mouth with a damp cloth. She did all of this with a smile and a voice as tender as Mother Teresa's. She was not only a credit to her profession but a credit to all humanity, and it was quite obvious that she not only loved what she was doing, but she was an experienced soul.

I could no longer sleep, so Sherri encouraged me to eat a pack of peanut butter and cheese crackers. I nibbled on a cracker, but the smell and taste of peanut butter alone prevented me from eating more. To my surprise, the elderly woman, after her sickness subsided, ate several crackers. Apparently the medical community felt as though peanut butter and cheese crackers could soothe the stomach and make chemotherapy more tolerable. Maybe there is some validity to their power, but the peanut butter reminded me of my first obstruction after surgery, so I wasn't about to eat one.

I glanced around the room briefly at the other four chemotherapy patients. I wondered how each one had arrived at this destination. Was it hereditary? Had they neglected their doctors' advice to have a colonoscopy as I had done, or were they simply sufferers of this unrelenting disease? It didn't really matter. We were all in the treatment room for the same reason: we had made the decision to fight cancer and we wanted to live no matter what or how much we had to endure.

Sherri and Michelle worked nonstop; their movements were managed and fluid, like a skilled surgeon's. I listened to the beep of the machines. From a small table near the cocktail counter a middle-aged man who walked with a cane waited for Michelle to remove his 5-FU pump; the familiar sound was the same *click-clunk* that I would be hearing for the next two days.

I closed my eyes and for some unknown reason found myself hovering above the room observing the drama, including my own. I appeared older than I remembered when I had shaved earlier in the morning, but, just like the others, I looked at peace. I watched for almost an hour, although it seemed like only seconds, until the beeping of my own machine brought me back to the reality of the treatment room.

Sherri unhooked my IV and flushed the port and then hooked me to the 5-FU pump; *click-clunk, click-clunk.* I waited in the recliner for another fifteen minutes before Debbie arrived. She thanked Michelle and Sherri and we left the medical center. She was eager to know how the treatment went and I responded as best as I could, but I was spent. Fatigue had overtaken my body; it took all of my energy just to hold my head erect. I felt like a puppet without a puppeteer.

I slept on the couch most of the afternoon and awoke to more fatigue coupled with nausea. Debbie encouraged me to eat a cup of chicken soup and a small piece of apple fritter, but I could hardly chew. My cheeks cramped, and along with the nausea and fatigue, my fingertips had gone completely numb. I felt miserable, even sorry for myself, and there was nothing Debbie could do to make me feel better. But, as usual, she had an answer. An hour later I received a phone call, not just any phone call, but one of the most important of my life from a woman who would help me through the long and tough road ahead.

CHAPTER 10

The Phone Call

HER NAME was Mary.

I had met and talked with her at a holiday party thrown by Debbie's co-workers the previous year. She was physically beautiful, in her early fifties with shoulder-length black hair, a wrinkle-free, sun-kissed complexion, and a bubbly smile that she could not contain, like an overflowing champagne flute. She had been diagnosed with inoperable pancreatic cancer three months earlier and was currently undergoing chemotherapy. And of course, it was Debbie who brought us together.

We talked a few minutes about Debbie and the reason for the call before I asked, "How are you feeling?"

"I've had better days," she said, and I could hear the fatigue in her voice. "Some days are better than others, but I'm hanging in there." She paused. "How are you handling the chemotherapy?"

"I had no idea what to expect, and it's tougher than I thought it would be," I replied. I tried to sound energetic, but I knew she could hear my fatigue as well. "The worst part so far has been the nausea. I don't want to eat anything except apple fritters, and right now I don't even want those."

She managed a quick laugh. "I know what you mean. I think everyone going through chemo has their own craving. This might sound a little weird, but the only thing that appeals to me is miso soup. And I never really liked it before I started chemo. And, get this, it has to be from the same restaurant or I won't eat it."

"I don't think it's weird at all. I totally understand." A long moment elapsed before I said, "Mary, I'm so sorry."

Her voice was strong. "It's okay, David. I've always been a fighter. I'm not about to let this beat me."

"But I feel guilty."

"Why on earth would you feel guilty?"

I hesitated, not knowing how to say what I was feeling, which really was guilt. "I was able to have surgery."

"There's no reason to feel guilty," she said. "You didn't cause it, but you're right. The worst part is living each day knowing that cancer is eating me alive, and there is nothing surgically that can be done."

I didn't know what to say. Here I was complaining about having a tough time with chemotherapy and the woman I was talking to had inoperable cancer and the heavy doses of chemotherapy she was taking could only offer, at best, a 4–5 percent chance of saving her life. Each time I had cancer, it was operable, so I can't imagine what she felt. She must have sensed my thoughts because she said, "There are those who have survived pancreatic cancer and I intend to add my name to that list." I knew there were tears in her eyes, but her voice was strong and determined. "I will never give up. And I want you to make me a promise right now that you will never quit. Never!"

It was all I could do to hold back tears. "If I don't wake up in the morning, it won't be because I refused to fight. I give you my word that I'll never quit, and I know you won't either."

"It's nice to be able to talk to someone who understands," she said, "and I hope we can talk often."

"I would like that," I replied.

"Then let's make this a habit."

"Thanks for calling," I said. "It means a lot to me."

I clicked the phone off and sat in silence. The spiritual connection with Mary was instant and overwhelming. At the moment, I felt as though God had sent an angel to watch over me, an angel who would be with me until I drew my last breath on this earth. Little did I know that's exactly what He'd done.

CHAPTER 11

Increasing Side Effects

THE NEXT day was physically and emotionally difficult for me, but I kept the conversation with Mary in my thoughts and willed myself to eat. Forcing food down my throat when there was a knot as big as a baseball in my stomach and a metallic taste in my mouth was not an easy task, especially knowing the regurgitation monster was close by. That was another reason I had such high praise and respect for those professionals and family members who take care of us and endure the daily smell of chemicals and death—something I have never been able to stomach, not even as that invincible twenty-year-old in Vietnam.

I've always done well under pressure when dealing with injuries to myself and others, including all the broken bones and bloody gashes my children sustained while they were growing up. But there was never food involved when taking care of those situations. I can't imagine eating a piece of my mother's fried chicken while holding a compress to a gushing two-inch gash, or eating a bag of chips while watching a dislocated bone being set, or, the worst case scenario, devouring a sandwich while looking at dead or mangled soldiers. Perhaps that sounds too bizarre or too outlandish, but it's something I've witnessed and will never forget, something that confronted me soon after I arrived in Vietnam.

I had been in-country for almost two months, mostly pulling guard duty and working in personal effects in a compound called Camp Red Ball on the outskirts of Saigon. Then, whether it was a promotion or punishment from the effects of my smart mouth, I was assigned to the team that retrieved the personal effects of soldiers killed in action from the morgue. I wasn't looking forward to the assignment, but I had little choice.

I suppose my first trip to the morgue was sort of an induction—like the final night of pledging for a college fraternity. We loaded a deuce-and-a-half—a two-and-one-half-ton utility truck—with personal effects, and then I was told by the buck sergeant in command to make a final check to make sure everything had been loaded. I was new and eager to please my superiors, hoping for a promotion to Private First Class (PFC), so I jumped out of the rear of the truck and checked all of the tents and hooches.

They left me.

I stood in the dirt road for ten minutes outside the large one-story concrete building that was used as a morgue waiting for my three comrades to come back and pick me up. It was a joke. I got it. But I wasn't laughing.

I reluctantly gave up my wait and walked through the series of tents and hooches that had held the personal effects we had loaded. Each structure had an armed guard at each entrance and exit twenty-four-seven. I should have known at that time, from the snickers from the guards, that I was just another notch on the sergeant's belt. Then I entered the morgue. What I saw made me as sick as I had ever been.

There were bodies everywhere; some where whole, some were cut up, and some were masses of twisted and charred flesh. The smell of death was everywhere. I saw one soldier eating a sandwich while working on an unrecognizable body. Then I saw others doing the same thing: eating. I ran for the door and threw up everything in my stomach; and then I dry heaved for ten minutes.

An hour later, after calming down by breathing deeply over and over again while standing in fresh air and washing my face at least five times with cold water, I lobbied a ride back to Camp Red Ball in an MP jeep.

When I arrived, it seemed as though the entire compound was laughing at me. Everywhere I went there were snorts and teasing and comments like, "Did you find the snipe?" and "Welcome to Vietnam."

I returned to the morgue the next day, and the next. Each time I lost my stomach, but I didn't care. I was beginning to feel something that was beyond dealing with the dead and getting sick. There was a spiritual connectedness all around me, and I felt the reassurance of being alive.

I made the trip to the morgue every day for the next two months. Each trip was the same. I helped load the deuce-and-a-half with personal effects to be shipped back to loved ones in the States, and then I remained behind, emptied my stomach, and helped out in the morgue. I always hitched a ride back to the compound with the same MP. After the first week no one at Camp Red Ball laughed at me. And there were no more comments. Instead, there was an occasional pat on the back. I didn't need the recognition, but it felt good to be acknowledged by others.

Regardless of the reason I stayed at the morgue, I'm glad I made the choice. Obviously, my physical being didn't agree with my decision, but my spirit rejoiced, and I know that today I am a better person.

On Wednesday I had the 5-FU pump removed, and on Friday I had another progress appointment with Dr. Rosen. After two full treatments, the side effects had increased: fatigue, nausea, cramping in my cheeks, numbness in my fingers, and now tingling in my toes. And Debbie had noticed irregularities with my cognitive functioning: confusion, concentration, memory, and multitasking. Yet Dr. Rosen was quite pleased with the results of the first two treatments.

With Oxaliplatin and 5-FU shooting through my system, I was in somewhat of a stupor the entire first week of each treatment and oftentimes found myself moving in slow motion. I was sluggish with my response to questions and was actually confused over certain words. I couldn't understand why a tree was called a tree and why it was spelled the way it was. It could have been called sunshine, which would have been fine with me. The same was true with the word hat, and I didn't understand why it was supposed to be worn on the head. Why not wear it on a shoulder? I also had trouble pronouncing and writing the letter J and the number five. And although I would never admit it until now, on occasion I struggled with the name Debbie, the very name of the person I love so much and who had helped me through the entire process. The name was foreign and difficult to pronounce. Why? I haven't a clue. But what was more perplexing was that I knew it was happening and couldn't control it. It was much like, I believe, a paraplegic willing his or her legs to move, yet without so much as a twitch of motion. But the second week without the chemical cocktails, I was sharper and less confused.

Also during the initial week of each treatment, my concentration took the same holiday as my taste buds. Focusing on a task and sticking to it was impossible. I love sports and look forward to reading the sports section of our local newspaper while eating breakfast each day, but in that initial week, I could not read its entirety in one sitting and would return time and time again throughout the day to finish. Oftentimes, when I remembered and returned, I would also find a plate of half-eaten grits and eggs. I've always had trouble hearing high-pitched noises, but during this time my ears were like radar; they picked up everything, and everything distracted me. I could be in the middle of a conversation with Debbie and suddenly not hear a word she was saying because someone walked by. And then for no reason at all I would just walk away from her and begin doing something else. This is not selective hearing, as some would suggest of their mates. Rather it was a mental lapse, as if my brain had short-circuited, leaving too large of a gap for the signal to hurdle. I left water running in the sink, put butter in the cabinet instead of returning it to the refrigerator, and tried to wash clothes in the dryer.

My short-term memory was a stowaway with my concentration, but my long-term remembrance of Mickey Mantle's and Babe Ruth's baseball statistics were always on the tip of my tongue. Debbie could ask me to do something and I would agree, and then I would walk into the next room to oblige her, become distracted with a leaf that had fallen off a plant, and walk to the screen door and stare at the huge coral tree in front of our house. I'm the first to agree that men sometimes have trouble listening to and understanding what their wives say and tend to only hear what they choose, and if asked to repeat what was just said, we oftentimes get it wrong. This was totally different. During the first week of chemotherapy, it was difficult to process and remember what was said. Although the second week was usually much better, my cognitive functioning fell short of what it was before the chemotherapy.

Multitasking during chemotherapy was like trying to whistle with a mouthful of crackers. (Ask any married woman and she will most likely say that men are confused much of the time, that their concentration and memory are selective, and that they absolutely cannot multitask. It's as though we live our entire married lives in a chemotherapy fog.) Multitasking was never a priority for me; I would rather concentrate on one item at a time, finish it, and go on from there. However, during chemotherapy I didn't have much of a choice. It was difficult to tie my shoes and talk at the same time.

It was disheartening to experience decreased cognitive functioning the first week of each treatment. However, it helped to know I would be a little more in control the second week. But then it was just as hard knowing that I would have to start all over again on Monday. I was praying that when chemotherapy was over, I would return to normal—whatever that is. What I was experiencing was foreign and frightening, and I had no idea how to deal with it. I've always liked being in control, and it's frustrating when that control is taken away. I sometimes think that the early stages of Alzheimer's disease must be similar, which reminds me of Ben.

Ben was in his early sixties when he was diagnosed with Alzheimer's. He was seventy when I first met him at the adult day care center I directed after I first moved to Southern California. He was physically healthy and had played pro baseball in the late 1940s. He was happy, active, and very cooperative in all of the activities at the center, and though most of the time he made little sense when he communicated, he loved to hear me talk about baseball.

At the mere mention of a baseball game, bat, glove, or ball, he beamed with pride and remembrance of the game he loved. Although his words were confused and broken, his smile and enthusiasm captivated me.

One day, in 1993, as we sat together talking at the adult day center, having a conversation about baseball that made no sense whatsoever, he paused and stared blankly at me for what seemed like an hour, yet it was only a moment. He shot me a half smile and then said, "I know what's happening to me, but I can't stop it."

I was floored. I wanted to run and tell everyone I knew in the medical profession what had happened, but I quickly dismissed the idea. How could I prove it? I couldn't. I might be looked upon by my peers and society as mentally deficient myself. So I've keep it within me all of these years.

Ben never said anything else that even resembled a complete sentence, at least not in my presence. His words were always scrambled, but I knew his soul was completely intact and willing his body to perform. How could I know this? When he stared at me and then spoke, he did so with his soul. And I listened.

I talked to Mary on Friday evening, but our conversation was short. She was unable to keep anything in her stomach and was weak and tired. Though we talked little, just hearing her voice gave me strength. We talked again on Monday evening and she was better. Her doctor had changed her chemotherapy and the dosage. She was eating and in good spirits, and we shared a few laughs.

I, too, was able to eat, though my taste buds were still somewhere south of the border. Each day without 5-FU flowing through my system, the nausea subsided, though the other side effects remained.

Mary and I talked on Thursday and again on Sunday, and both conversations were upbeat and fun, as if we were old friends sharing past episodes. "Do you remember the party last Christmas when Debbie asked us if we knew what the thin strings under a banana peel were called?"

I laughed as I recalled the hilarious chit-chat between friends, chit-chat after a couple glasses of wine.

"I told her they were potassium strips," Mary continued. "Everyone thought that was a funny answer, but when Debbie called them sniglets, we roared with laughter. She said that everything that didn't have a name is called a sniglet.

"I remember," I said, laughing with her. It was so good to hear her full of life. It was like listening to the Mary I knew who did not have a deadly cancer growing inside her.

She wished me good luck on Monday as I started another round of chemotherapy, and I promised to call her and let her know how it went.

CHAPTER 12

Birthday Chemotherapy

I DREADED Monday morning, October 16. It was the day before my fifty-ninth birthday, and, after only two treatments, I was battered and weak, like wood timbers of a hurricane-ravaged pier. I wanted nothing more to do with chemotherapy. It was difficult handling a week of nausea, fatigue, continuing side effects, and cognitive impairments, and then recuperating only enough to turn around and do it again. But I had decided I would never give up. I had too much to live for, and now that Mary was in my life, I had promised her that I would remain strong as well. I wanted to be there for her. I also realized that no matter how difficult my problems, many others were in far worse situations. I saw it during each of my treatments. And what about the children in cancer hospitals who have never known a day without suffering and chemotherapy? They were the real heroes. They were the ones with more courage than the cowardly lion could ever hope to have.

My Oxaliplatin treatment was uneventful. John took me and Debbie picked me up. I slept most of the afternoon on the couch with the *click-clunk* of the 5-FU pump, forced a can of soup down for dinner, and went to bed early.

Tuesday morning was my birthday. I awoke feeling so sick, I stayed in bed. By noon I felt better and made it to the couch. Debbie fixed a steak dinner, which I couldn't eat, and Amanda joined us and brought a cherry pie. Birthday or not, I didn't feel good—and I could not put on an act. Debbie and Amanda understood and didn't push me. They knew I loved them and was thankful that they cared.

Mary called and wished me a happy birthday. Just hearing from her improved my morale, but what I heard next was difficult. She had been to the doctor, and the news wasn't good. The change in chemotherapy she had received over the past week and a half had allowed her to eat more and keep it down—she only weighed a hundred and ten pounds—but it had done nothing to arrest the cancer. In fact, her oncologist thought the cancer had spread even more and she had begun the same heavy doses of chemotherapy as before.

I knew she wasn't telling me everything, and I wasn't going to ask her. But I could read between the lines. I later learned from Debbie that hospice had already been contacted.

Moments after I hung up, Amanda and Debbie came into the living room carrying a piece of cherry pie with a candle and presents. It was a wonderful gesture from two people who love me unconditionally. I found that it took all of my energy to blow out just one candle and was thankful they didn't saturate the entire pie with fifty-nine. Cherry pie is my favorite, so I ate a small piece, but it was the gifts that touched my heart.

Amanda's gift was an iPod that she had loaded with songs from the late 50s and early 60s, and Debbie gave me earphones that blocked most exterior noise. Their intent was that my favorite songs would help me with the anxiety while having my Monday morning cocktail. Not only were they right, but the solidarity and music seemed to help with the nausea. How? Again, I haven't a clue. What they had done not only displayed kindness, compassion, and love (not to mention complete ingenuity) but it was something I will never forget. It was one of the most thoughtful things anyone has ever done for me. On that day, they made contact with my soul, and I am a better person because of it.

I went to sleep that night listening to music on my new iPod thinking of what was happening in Mary's life and how lucky I was. As sick as I had been most of the day, it turned out to be one of my most memorable birthdays.

I called Mary on Thursday night, but her caregiver told me she was too ill to talk. I called again on Saturday with the same results, but I was surprised by a call from her on Sunday afternoon. Her voice was weak as she said, "I can't eat and I'm down to one hundred pounds. I have a doctor's appointment tomorrow morning. He told me on Friday that we could try something else, so I'm going to be optimistic."

"That's great," I said, although I was sure my tone wasn't as enthusiastic as it should have been. "Remember what we talked about? Well, I'm holding you to it. You're never going to give up. Never."

"I remember."

I suddenly realized our roles were reversed. She had been supporting and encouraging me for almost six weeks, and much of the time without reciprocation, but now it was my turn. "Are you still eating the miso soup you like?"

"I can't eat much of anything," she said.

"I'd be happy to go to that Japanese restaurant in the shopping center and get you a to-go container."

"No," she said, "but thanks."

"Please try to eat," I said. "I'll be thinking about you and sending you lots of love tomorrow. Good luck."

I hung up and leaned my head back on the chair and stared at the ceiling fan, watching it slowly turn for the better part of an hour. I was entering the part of the treatment cycle where I began feeling better. I still had the same side effects, and there were two new ones: my body itched as if I had walked naked through a patch of poison oak and I was experiencing periods of diarrhea.

"Not related," Dr Rosen informed me, but I knew different. We all know our bodies better than anyone, better than doctors, psychics, and loved ones, and it is up to each of us to understand and act upon what we feel inside.

My appetite was returning, so I went to the refrigerator and broke a cold apple fritter in half. I was actually hungry, yet I felt guilty thinking of Mary. But I had to eat if I was going to beat this. I was going to be there for a dear friend, no matter how long it took.

CHAPTER 13

Chemotherapy 4 and 5

I WAS ready for the fourth round of chemotherapy Monday morning, October 30. John and I chatted for the first ten minutes after my cocktail was ready, and then I turned on my iPod and sank into oblivion. The routine was the same: cocktail, flush the port, hook up the 5-FU pump. It was also the same routine for John: watch me until I was in another realm, wait twenty to thirty minutes in the waiting room, check on me, then leave. Is it any wonder why I love this guy?

Debbie picked me up at twelve thirty. She was shocked when I said, "Why don't we go out to lunch?"

A smile lit her face, one I hadn't seen since my old adversary had returned. "Where would you like to go?"

"I want a hamburger. How about that little place down by the harbor?"

Debbie's smile grew. "My treat."

I was already nauseous from the 5-FU but managed to keep the burger in my stomach. When we arrived home, I did not collapse on the sofa or take a nap; instead, Debbie and I sat on the patio for an hour and talked, and then we went for a walk around the park. It took every ounce of energy I had, but I was determined to recapture control of my life.

Though I wasn't hungry, I ate a small portion of linguini with vegetable sauce and salad for dinner. Again I willed myself to keep it down, and it worked, although the regurgitation monster was continually lodged in my throat.

After dinner I called Mary. Her doctor's appointment had gone well. The new treatment appeared to be working, and she had gone to lunch with her caregiver. Of course she had miso soup. She was weak and still only one hundred pounds, yet there was hope hanging on every word. Needless to say, her news lifted my spirits immediately, and for the first time since I was told of her inoperable condition, I felt as though we would one day share a cancer survivor celebration.

I had another appointment with Dr. Rosen on Friday. My red and white blood cell counts were finally in the good range, yet all of the side effects still persisted. A new one had surfaced as well: at times, especially during the 5-FU treatment, my face flushed as if I had been exposed to a bright, hot sun for several hours.

"Not related," Dr. Rosen said again, and I immediately ignored her statement. I didn't tell her about the cognitive difficulties I was having. Debbie and I agreed that she would probably disregard my claim of confusion and forgetfulness and attribute it to the aging process.

Friday night was party time. Debbie's birthday and retirement were on the same day, and there must have been sixty of her closest friends and colleagues dancing to her favorite music: Motown, especially Diana Ross and Marvin Gaye. It was a very special night for her. She had been taking care of me for two and a half months and had little time for herself, so it was good to see her let her hair down—and can she ever let her hair down. I had forgotten how beautiful she was and how much she enjoyed dancing, and watching her delighted my soul. The night belonged to her.

I was still somewhat nauseous but did the best I could to stay upbeat. I mostly kept to the side of the dance floor in a cushioned chair, occasionally talking to those who acknowledged me. It brought tears to my eyes when she included me in several slow dances and whispered in my ear, "I love you."

I hadn't talked to Mary since Monday and figured no news was good news. I called her on Wednesday and she was a real Chatty Cathy. Her voice was strong and she had gained a few pounds. "Why don't you ask your doctor for a B-12 shot?" she said after we had discussed fatigue.

"You think that might help?"

"It certainly can't hurt," she said. "I know several others with cancer who highly recommended it to me."

So Wednesday morning I called Dr. Stone's office and scheduled an appointment for one o'clock. The shot took only a few seconds, but he took extra time to talk with me. I told him about the chemotherapy and the side effects, but other than the B-12 shot, there didn't appear to be anything he could do to help. He thought some of the side effects I explained were due to nerve damage. It was reassuring just talking to him, and he wanted me to keep him informed of my progress.

I talked to Mary again on Sunday. She was still feeling good and had gained another pound. Things were looking great for both of us. My outlook for the next treatment was optimistic, not that I was looking forward to it, but I had finally decided I was going to fight the sickness with every ounce of my total being. Actually, I had already made that decision, but it doesn't hurt to rededicate oneself. (It's similar to a pregame routine by a pitcher before he takes the mound. More often than not, being mentally prepared to pitch usually results in a win. I think the same can be said when facing surgery or chemotherapy.) It added to my confidence and my emotional stability. And my concern for Mary had turned to optimism. For the first time, I believed that she was really going to make it.

I did realize that the jury was still out for a total recovery for both of us. I have witnessed the eye of a hurricane and the calm before a storm many times in my life, but I had a good feeling and I was going to ride it as long as I could.

John the Faithful again took me for my Oxaliplatin cocktail on November 13. It had become a ritual now. Although Debbie was retired, I knew he would accompany me throughout the entire treatment process. I didn't realize how much that meant until it was all over; it was an act of love on his part. I will always value his friendship, and he'll always have a special place in my heart.

I believe that a strong support group beyond family members is a large part of surviving cancer and chemotherapy. Oftentimes friends want no part of sickness. Whether it reveals that they aren't really friends or that they just can't handle the situation doesn't really matter. If we can't give of ourselves during difficult situations, what good is it to give under all of the right circumstances? That is why I consider John to be an exceptional human being.

I wasn't as chipper in the evening after my morning cocktail as I was during the last treatment, but I ate as much as I could and kept it down. Remaining active, which included frequent walks with Debbie, seemed to help with the nausea, or maybe it was the fact that exercise kept my mind off the sickness.

Wednesday midmorning, with the 5-FU still *click-clunking* through my veins, I had several sharp pains in my chest near the location of the port. I immediately dropped to the couch and sucked in a long breath. The pain subsided and I was up again, getting ready to go to the treatment room to have the pump removed. The pain hit again and took my breath away, but it was over quickly, so I thought nothing more of it. I didn't even mention it to Michelle or Sherri.

I felt better on Thursday and called Mary. My heart broke when she told me the news wasn't good. Again, the new treatment, though it had allowed her to eat and become more active, wasn't working as her doctor had hoped, so he placed her on a larger oral dose of the original chemotherapy. She was sick and had lost a couple of pounds, and the optimism I had recently heard in her voice was gone.

I felt so helpless when I clicked the phone off that I wanted to yell and curse every cancer cell that had ever existed. Debbie had gone to LAX to pick up Linda, her best friend from high school who was coming for a visit, so I allowed the floodgates to open and I let everything go. I cursed and sobbed for Mary, for myself, and for everyone—past and present—who had cancer and had to undergo chemotherapy, and for those who would endure it in the future. I cried for my mother (though her cancer was most likely self-induced by smoking) who died at age fifty-five from bone cancer that had spread from her lungs. And I cried for all of those dedicated family, friends, and medical personnel who have given of themselves to care for a cancer patient.

I cried until I had no more tears to give, and then I sat just staring at a blank television screen. Sometimes life isn't fair. Sure, my year in Vietnam, my own cancer at an early age that robbed me of my boyhood dream of playing pro baseball, and the unexpected death of my mother were proof enough. But knowing

Mary was slipping away seemed more unfair than anything I had ever experienced. At that very moment, without even an extra thought, I would gladly have traded my life for hers.

On Saturday I had a few more sharp pains in my chest, again near the area of the port, but they subsided quickly and I gave it no more thought. I called Mary several times, but her caregiver relayed the message that she was too sick to talk.

I was ashamed of my pity meltdown on Thursday, but it was also beneficial to my spirit. Sometimes I guess it's just good to get it all out. I was determined more than ever to remain strong and fight my way through this. If Mary couldn't fight, then I would do it for her. After all, she was my angel, and now I was hers.

CHAPTER 14

Chemotherapy 6

JOHN TOOK me for my biweekly cocktail on November 27 and then picked me and my 5-FU pump buddy up at twelve forty-five. Debbie and Linda were at lunch celebrating Linda's birthday, so rather than dropping me off at the house, John took me to lunch at Ball Street Café. I was still pretty doped up from the Ativan that accompanied the Oxaliplatin, so nausea from the 5-FU had not kicked in.

After a hot bowl of potato soup on the patio, John dropped me off at home. As the kind and caring person he is, he wanted to wait with me until Debbie arrived, but I assured him I was fine and would just take a nap. I woke when Debbie and Linda arrived home around three o'clock and was hit by a wave of nausea. I managed half of an apple fritter for dinner, but I couldn't keep it down.

Debbie encouraged me to call Mary around seven. I didn't want to move or talk for fear of being sick again, so I asked her to make the call for me. On other occasions Debbie had talked with Mary either before or after our conversation, so it wasn't entirely a surprise request.

After ten minutes of listening, I more than understood the entire conversation with Mary's caregiver. Hospice was now involved, taking care of Mary and preparing her for what was inevitably going to happen. Though I didn't want to believe it, I knew the end for Mary was getting closer with each passing day.

The following morning I woke at six thirty with severe chest pain. I woke Debbie, and then remained in bed while she phoned Dr. Rosen's office. Of course no one was there, so she left a message with the answering service for Dr. Rosen to return the call.

By now Linda was up and aware of what was happening. She was Debbie's height and thin with a distinct *Fargo* accent, and she wore her hair in a stylish brown bob. She had been in the medical field as a medical assistant for over thirty years with a private physician and knew the right questions to ask. "Do you have numbness or pain in your arms?"

I told her no and explained that I had experienced the pain before and that it didn't feel as if it was related to my heart. And just as I said it, the pain subsided.

Debbie pleaded with me to go to the emergency room, but I wanted no part of a hospital. I just wanted to rest until Dr. Rosen called.

By seven thirty the pain was back, not as severe as before, but enough to finally make me realize something was wrong and that it wasn't going to take care of itself. At eight, Dr. Rosen still had not called. I wasn't going to the hospital, but I agreed to go to Dr. Stone's office. We arrived at eight thirty, and the nurse took me in immediately for an EKG. There was no evidence of a heart attack.

I wasn't surprised that the EKG was normal. Dr. Stone suggested it could be a malfunction with the Portacath, so he sent me to the Conchita hospital for X-rays.

Linda remained at the house waiting for the call from Dr. Rosen, and then gave Dr. Rosen Debbie's cell number. Debbie's phone rang just as we pulled into the hospital parking lot. She explained the past several hours and Dr. Rosen recommended I immediately turn off the 5-FU pump, have the X-rays, request a copy from the radiologist, and then get to her office at once.

The X-rays, after the pump had been restarted and dye had been injected into the port, seemed to take forever. It was one o'clock before we arrived at Dr. Rosen's office. She took the 5-FU pump and gave it to Michelle to check for malfunction and then scanned the X-rays and radiologist's report that the Portacath was functioning properly.

Although I had had no chest pain for the past several hours, she insisted that I check into University Hospital for tests that she would set up at once with a cardiologist, so two hours later I was in a semi-private room waiting for Dr. O'Sullivan, a cardiologist in his late forties with black wavy hair who dressed like an Ivy League graduate.

Debbie had been with me the entire day and helped explain everything that had happened.

"You must have some thought as to what is going on," she said.

Dr. O'Sullivan flashed a quick smile. "I have an idea, but why don't we wait and see what the tests reveal."

I was tired, hungry, and wanted some answers. "That's not fair, doc. I don't expect you to make a diagnosis without further tests, but at least point us in the general direction of what the hell is happening."

He lost his smile. "You'll be the first to know as soon as the tests are over."

I glared at him. "Are you good at what you do?"

"David!" Debbie exclaimed.

Dr. Sullivan's preppy smile was back. "I'm the one you want in your corner."

I suddenly loved this guy. "Okay, let's do the tests."

The following morning I woke early, not by choice, but to the clanging of medicine carts, nurses hurrying about their duties, and the growl in my stomach. Debbie had not remained overnight with me since I was on no pain meds or seeing wallpaper-camouflaged urinals. I didn't even have an IV hooked to my forearm.

I was allowed nothing to eat until after the tests, so I watched the guy next to me—a burly cop who was recovering from shoulder surgery—eat a hospital breakfast that somehow looked like it was from a gourmet restaurant. At eight o'clock I had an X-ray with dye added through the Portacath, the same procedure done the day before at the hospital in Conchita. I decided Dr. O'Sullivan didn't believe the out-of-town radiologist. The next test was at nine thirty, a treadmill procedure I had never had before with wires taped to my chest leading to at least five different machines.

Everything was proceeding smoothly until eleven fifteen when I was scheduled for a PET scan. When I saw the machine and the technicians explained the procedure, I had a full-blown panic attack. I had to leave the room and get fresh air; I had to move, I had to pace. Debbie wasn't with me for the test. She had used the time to run a few errands, but a nurse reached her on her cell phone and she was at the hospital in ten minutes. Debbie could calm a storm, and, as usual, she calmed me—although it was not enough to make me submit to the terrifying machine.

An hour later, after more pacing and two milligrams of Ativan, I was able to endure the test, but only with Debbie standing by me whispering calming stories about our snorkeling adventures in Virgin Gorda, British Virgin Islands, as the menacing machine whirred back and forth over my chest. If I live to be a hundred, I could never even come close to thanking her enough for the many times she has rescued me from my own fears.

When I returned to my room the cop was eating a hamburger and french fries. But lunchtime had come and gone, and when I asked about having yummy hospital food, I was told that Dr. O'Sullivan wanted to review the test results before I ate anything.

"Is he reviewing them now?" I asked.

"I don't know," replied a brunette, middle-aged shift nurse.

"What time does he usually come by?" I asked again.

"Most of the doctors make their rounds between four and six," she replied.

I glanced at Debbie. She shrugged and smiled. "Sorry, dear, you're just going to have to wait."

And wait I did. Dr. O'Sullivan arrived at four thirty with good news. My heart was strong and there was no evidence that I had suffered a heart attack. However, he did suggest that just above the port's catheter the left internal jugular vein had most likely collapsed under the bombardment of 5-FU. "A very rare side effect," he explained, "but without the 5-FU, the vein has returned to its normal size and is functioning properly."

Debbie and I had a ton of questions, the first being, "Why?" He began explaining when Dr. Rosen entered, as if on cue, and took his place. We thanked him and he left, and I again asked, "Why did this happen?"

Dr. Rosen skipped and danced around the question and never really explained it, most likely because she didn't understand it either. However, she did say it was a potential side effect that rarely occurred, and when it did, it was only in less than 5 percent of those on 5-FU intravenously. (It would have been good to know that there was a chance of this happening before I started chemotherapy.)

"Will this affect his heart in the future?" Debbie asked.

"It shouldn't," Dr. Rosen replied, "but there are no guarantees of any kind with chemotherapy. And remember, this has not affected his heart, just the vein."

I wanted to ask, "How can a vein collapse and then return to normal size without any damage? Wouldn't that area become a weak link?" But I held my tongue.

Dr. Rosen answered the fusillade of questions we threw at her. Finally, we asked, "What's next?"

"Well, we know that you can handle the Oxaliplatin. It's the 5-FU that is in question. We'll stop the chemotherapy for three to four weeks and let you get stronger. Then we'll resume the Oxaliplatin, and I want you to give 5-FU a try in pill form." I could no longer hold my tongue and was quick with the next question. "If it's the 5-FU causing my vein to collapse, wouldn't it be the same in pill form?"

"Not necessarily," Dr. Rosen answered. "This 5-FU dosage will dissolve in your stomach and travel through your system in lower concentration than intravenously. I see no reason why we shouldn't be able to resume the schedule we were on."

I suddenly remembered Mary and the large doses she had taken. She was constantly nauseated and couldn't keep anything in her stomach. I wondered how she was doing, and then I realized that she would jump at the chance to try something new.

Debbie had been standing by the hospital bed holding my hand during the entire conversation. She nodded, and then I agreed, "Okay."

"Good," said Dr. Rosen. "Now let's get you out of here."

It took an hour to check out of the hospital. We decided to start the next treatment on Tuesday, January 2, 2007, but I was to schedule an appointment with Dr. Rosen in her office on Friday, December 29, 2006.

I was lucky there had been no permanent damage to my heart, but when I thought of Mary, the damage was insurmountable. I cared so much for her. I wanted her to live, and I wanted her to be as lucky as I was to have another chance. I wanted her to always be around so I could talk to someone who understood how I felt, but unless a miracle happened, my friend wasn't going to make it.

CHAPTER 15

Mary

A MONTH can seem like forever when, in actuality, it represents only a sliver of time. Without the chemotherapy, I was getting stronger every day. My appetite had returned and I had gained almost ten pounds during the month of December. Despite the lingering side effects, I was back to a somewhat normal life. Debbie even commented that I appeared to be mentally sharper the last couple of weeks. And I was.

The confusion I had experienced wasn't there, or if it was, it wasn't as pronounced. The words "tree" and "hat" made perfect sense, the letter J and number five were easily pronounced and written. And, thank goodness, the name "Debbie" was as familiar as eating breakfast.

My concentration had definitely improved. I could read the entire sports page and finish my eggs and grits in one sitting, and I could actually carry on a conversation with Debbie and finish it, and then understand what had taken place. There was no leaving the water running while going outside, no butter in cabinets, and the dryer was not used as the washing machine.

My short-term memory was better, but I was still having trouble remembering what I had done the day before at the snap of a finger. Eventually I would recall the previous day's events, but it seemed as though I had to search my brain longer than normal to find what I was looking for.

And as for multitasking, yes, I can do it, but I still prefer doing one thing a time, finishing it, and moving on to the next item.

I talked to Mary only twice before Christmas. The other times I called she was too weak to get out of bed, where she now spent a great deal of her time. Hospice had been helping with her care as her condition deteriorated, but she still had a few good days.

Debbie managed to talk her into letting us visit, so on Wednesday the 27, two days after Christmas, we pulled into Mary's driveway on the east side of Santa Domingo at four o'clock in the afternoon.

Debbie and I hadn't seen Mary since early February, before she was diagnosed with pancreatic cancer, when we accepted her invitation to look at her backyard and barbeque area for ideas of our own. (I loved grilling out and usually did so two or three times a week, although over the past five months the barbeque area had become a ghost town. Mary's built-in Mexican-décor grill and counter area were unique and beautiful, and we now have a similar area on our patio.)

The physical Mary we knew did not answer the door. She had been a beautiful Mexican woman who brightened any room she entered, and I remember Debbie telling me how she uplifted everyone at work during stressful times. One of her favorite lines was, "Oh... my...God" before she proceeded to tell her version of a story.

The Mary who answered the door was weak and as thin as a strand of spaghetti, weighing maybe eighty-five pounds. Her face was wrinkled from the severe weight loss and her black hair was crew-cut short, but as I looked into her eyes, I saw the beauty of the woman I had grown to love over the phone.

She welcomed us and introduced us to her caregiver, who took the quart of miso soup we stopped and purchased at a Japanese restaurant, and then Debbie and I sat on the couch. Conversation was awkward at first, but after a few minutes, I felt as comfortable as if I were at home talking with Debbie or at the treatment center listening to John.

We spoke briefly about how she was feeling. Debbie and I listened earnestly, but it was obvious that she didn't want to talk about her illness. She wanted to know all about me, how I was doing, and if I was still writing. So the conversation switched to me.

I told her the same things we had already discussed on the phone; the episode with the 5-FU and the collapse of the jugular vein and the next round of chemotherapy, and then I told her about a book I was writing.

I explained that the novel was about a physician who, after an accident and coma, came to understand how our souls develop spiritually and decided to teach others about God's love and how we must realize the importance of true love and forgiveness in order to progress. But the physician is challenged and ridiculed by local religious leaders, including his duplicitous televangelist father-in-law, and then he is framed for murder.

She loved the idea and appeared to understand why I wanted to write it. In fact, I knew she understood the part about spiritual development and true love and forgiveness. There was a maturity of her soul that was unmistakable, and I saw it in her eyes and heard it in her voice. Suddenly, I was ashamed to be talking so enthusiastically about writing a book, but I knew she was happy for me.

Debbie and I enjoyed a full hour with Mary; that was all she could handle. It seemed like only a few minutes, but I was thankful for any time I could spend with her. Debbie rose first and gave Mary a hug, and then I followed. When I took her in my arms, I hugged her tightly, yet gently, and felt the reality of her thinness. I could feel every rib. "I love you," I whispered so only she could hear.

"I love you, too," she whispered back.

I attempted to release the hug, but she held on a moment longer. That's the instant I felt an incredible energy source flowing from her. I kissed her on the cheek, and then, with a lump in my throat as large as a baseball, I stared into her soul. She was the most beautiful thing I had ever seen—her aura was cobalt blue—and I knew the love we had for one another was definitely the true love that God wants us to have.

Debbie and I walked to the car and got in without saying a word. Debbie drove, and when we were a block from Mary's house she pulled to the side of the road. Tears streamed over her cheeks.

"David, that wasn't Mary. That wasn't the woman who stopped by my office and cheered me up with an 'Oh...my...God.' I didn't even recognize her."

The lump was still in my throat. She was right; the physical Mary we knew existed now only in our hearts and our memories, but a better Mary had emerged, one who understood the meaning and beauty of life.

Debbie was sobbing. "Why does she look like that?"

Of course I knew the answer, but I had been just as shocked when I first saw Mary. I had seen it with my mother over three decades ago. From the moment she was diagnosed with cancer to the day she gave up was exactly three months. She went from a vibrant, attractive fifty-five-year-old woman to a fragile, thin, wrinkled old woman in a matter of months.

"The disease robs people of who they think they really are," I said.

"It's not fair."

"No, it's not," I said. "It's not fair that she and those who love her are suffering and I'm surviving."

Neither of us spoke for a long moment, and then Debbie turned to me. "I could use a drink. Let's go out to dinner."

I agreed wholeheartedly.

As Debbie drove, I wondered why two people can have a disease and one survives and the other…I couldn't say it. I refused to say it. I would cling to an old saying my mother had often used, "If you can think it, you can believe it. And if you can believe it, it can happen; even a miracle."

CHAPTER 16

Chemotherapy 7

I MET with Dr. Rosen on Friday morning, December 29, in her office. I had no chest pain, I had a healthy appetite, and I had gained at least ten pounds. My red and white blood cell counts were well within the normal range, so after a short question-and-answer session, she pronounced me fit for the next treatment. "There's no reason to wait any longer," she said. The woman was relentless, which was one of the things I liked best about her. But she took aggressiveness to a new level.

She gave me a prescription for the 5-FU pills, which I had filled at a local pharmacy. The bottle was wide and tall and loaded with enough poison to take me through the next six treatments. Looking at it made me nauseous, so I eagerly stuck it on the top shelf of the spice cabinet in our kitchen and quickly closed the door. I didn't want to see it until I absolutely had to, and Tuesday was coming soon enough. I wanted nothing more than to enjoy the weekend and New Year's Day.

Tuesday morning John took me to the medical center for my next Oxaliplatin cocktail. I had my headphones and iPod and was ready to face the monster. We arrived at nine o'clock and the treatment room was packed (even chemotherapy treatment centers took off for the holidays), so I had to wait thirty minutes for one of the recliners.

This is where John is so good. As a Korean and Vietnam War veteran, he had more stories than Uncle Remus and was able to keep my mind off the anxiousness of the morning. The stories worked, at least for a while, until one of the battles he described reminded me of the first meeting with my old nemesis.

It was early morning on January 31, 1968, and I was sleeping on a cot in what we called a hooch—a screened wood-frame building with a metal roof shaped like a Quonset hut.

Exploding mortars and rockets jolted me awake. I was disorientated for only a split second before grabbing my steel pot and running for the sand-bag bunker about twenty yards from the hooch.

The bunker was designed to hold about fifty soldiers, but there must have been at least seventy-five men already inside, all in underwear with steel helmets on their heads. We were as packed as a boatload of immigrants, but more soldiers kept pushing and shoving, cramming inside.

Bombs exploded like the Fourth of July. We heard yelling and screaming as others desperately sought a bunker they could squeeze into. Most were turned away and left exposed to the flying shrapnel.

The mortar attack was unrelenting and continued for the next six hours. It was always hot in Vietnam, but inside the bunker was like a sauna in mid-summer, and it had begun to stink of sweat and urine.

I've always been good under pressure and held it together in the bunker, but there were those who panicked and wanted out, which was not exactly a good choice with mortars exploding like a fireworks grand finale.

There were fights, and some were beaten and knocked unconscious.

At nine in the morning the barrage of mortars lessened. We fled the bunker, threw on our fatigues, grabbed our M-16s, and were quickly stationed in a narrow trench paralleling the chain-link surrounding our compound: Tent City B, Tan Son Nhut, South Vietnam.

We remained in the trench for three days. The only food we had were C-Rations, and there was little water for our canteens. Our objective was to stop the advancing Viet Cong that had taken over the ARVN—Army of the Republic of Vietnam—compound about five hundred yards from us. Between the ARVN compound and Tent City B was a large cemetery and open ground, but the VC were relentless. Their numbers were staggering, and surviving meant help from Cobra gunships—helicopters loaded with machine guns and rockets. The noise was deafening, but the results were remarkable. The gunships descended quickly and sprayed the cemetery with rockets. Even the VC were smart enough to back off.

At the end of the third day, intelligence informed our superiors that the VC had retreated. We were ecstatic, but we were also tired and hungry. Half of us returned to our hooches and the other half remained in the trenches—just in case.

Back at the hooch, I dropped my fatigues. The guy who bunked next to me—a heavyset Nebraska Cornhusker—saw blood on my neck. "You're wounded," he said. And then he yelled, "Get a medic!"

But I wasn't wounded. It was the mole on my neck, the reason for my first battle with malignant melanoma. It wasn't the first time the mole had bled, but this time—during the conflict that was later labeled "Tet Offensive," in which the Viet Cong and North Vietnamese Regulars simultaneously attacked every major city in South Vietnam and in which hundreds of U.S. troops and allies were killed, the mole had been severed. I had lost a lot of blood, and it was caked on my neck and collar.

I should have realized at the time that there was something wrong, but I was clueless. The mole grew back and I figured all was well, although it often bled when scratched or rubbed with a towel. I remained clueless throughout the remaining months of my Vietnam tour until I was safely back in the United States and my sergeant major ordered me to the hospital.

When my cocktail was ready, Michelle hooked me up. I put the headphones on and John left. Debbie arrived at twelve thirty, but my cocktail lasted until one o'clock.

The treatment room was still packed when we left. It felt weird not to have the 5-FU pump attached to my belt, with each *click-clunk* forcing the poison through my bloodstream.

For the first time in the last three weeks I wasn't hungry, but when we arrived home, Debbie made me a cup of soup. I ate it slowly, and then it was time.

I reluctantly opened the spice cabinet, vainly hoping someone had stolen the 5-FU pills. But they were right where I had left them. Following Dr. Rosen's instructions, I took four of the large tablets and swallowed them with a bottle of water. I had to take the same dosage two more times throughout the day and evening, four times on Wednesday, and then morning and noon on Thursday. Debbie sat next to me on the couch and we both waited to see if anything abnormal happened.

Nothing.

After fifteen minutes of waiting, I could hardly keep my eyes open, so I took a nap and slept until four thirty. When I woke, I wasn't nauseous. I couldn't believe it. I felt good and wanted something to eat.

My first thought was that Dr. Rosen was right. Perhaps the change in the way my body received and processed the 5-FU was right for me and would increase my chances of finishing all twelve of the treatments, which would also increase my chances of getting rid of any cancer cells still in my system. What I was feeling was almost too good to be true, and it was.

By eleven that night I was sicker than I had been at any time with the 5-FU pump. I slept little, continually making unscheduled trips to hug the porcelain god, and by eight thirty the following morning, just before I was to take the next dosage of pills, I experienced the first chest pain. I called Dr. Rosen's office and left a message. She returned my call at nine fifteen.

"Good morning, Mr. Yates," Dr. Rosen said. "I want you to stop the medication at once. You're finished with chemotherapy."

She referred me to her office coordinator and I scheduled an appointment for the following Tuesday. When I hung up the phone, my ears were still joyfully ringing with Dr. Rosen's words, "You're finished with chemotherapy." I was sick and my chest hurt, but I had a smile on my face.

Was it true? Was I totally finished with chemotherapy, or was something new waiting for me when I walked into her office?

I called Mary twice that week. The first time she was unable to talk. I wasn't given a reason, only that she was being cared for by hospice. The second call I connected with her, but the conversation was short.

"I'm not doing well," she replied.

I could hear it in her weak voice. She had given up. She had reached that spiritual plateau that everyone has when there is no longer any fight left in the physical body. There was nothing I could say or do, so I told her about my latest episode.

"I'm glad you're finally off the 5-FU," she said. "It's horrible."

"I know," I replied, "and I finally realize a little of what you've been going through. I don't know how you did it."

"I didn't do it very long," she said. "I couldn't."

"But you handled it much longer and better than I did. You're stronger than you think."

There was a long pause. "I'm tired, David. I have to hang up now."

"I want to come see you."

"I wouldn't want anyone to see me like this," she said.

"It doesn't matter, Mary. I need to see you."

Her words were slower and weaker than when we first began our conversation. "Let me get a little stronger first."

It must have been a real struggle for her to talk—I heard her gasp for a breath. "Okay," I said. "Get some rest."

I hung up realizing her time was close, but I had no idea that that was the last time I would ever talk to her.

Mary died two days later.

Of course I wasn't surprised to hear Debbie's words. The look on her face said it for her. "Mary passed away," she said, as a tear leaked from her eyes.

I was at the hospital with my mother when she died. The devastation I experienced then was overpowering to my spirit, but being able to talk with her up to the final minute was comforting and something I'm thankful for to this day. The devastation I felt over hearing that Mary had died was the same, and I was fortunate to have our phone conversations and the visit with her to comfort me.

I spent Monday afternoon as if I were in a trance, and then came the tears. I cried because I could never talk to my friend again. I cried because she had died and I was still alive, and I cried because I had lost one of the closest friends I had ever had. But how could that be? I had only really known her for four months, and most of our conversations had been on the phone.

I wondered if people sometimes felt strongly attached to others even if they hardly knew them, as if the bond was through a spiritual connection. That's how it was with

Mary. Though I don't exactly know how it works, I believe hers was another soul meant to be in my life.

I miss her. I'll always miss her, but she will forever be with me in my heart.

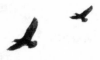

CHAPTER 17

No More Chemotherapy

"YOUR CHEMOTHERAPY is over," said Dr. Rosen as Debbie and I sat in her office Tuesday morning at nine thirty.

My heart was beating with profound joy, but my expression was as rigid as a Buckingham Palace guard's. I was afraid there was a "However" coming followed by, "We're going to try something different," so I simply nodded.

"How is that going to affect his chances for a complete recovery?" Debbie asked. "Does it increase the odds that the cancer will return?"

"I'm actually pleased that he finished half of the program," said Dr. Rosen. "The odds for a full recovery are much better than without any treatment."

"I understand that," said Debbie, who wasn't about to give up the question, "but wouldn't six more treatments be better?"

"Not necessarily," the doctor replied. "Not everyone makes it through the entire program. In fact, in your husband's case, I would consider finishing one-half to two-thirds of the treatment extremely good."

I was shocked. This information was news to me. I thought it was mandatory that I finish all of the treatments. I once saw two friends of a woman undergoing chemotherapy bring balloons for an intimate celebration during her last chemotherapy treatment. I thought it was a great display of kindness and compassion. It gave me something to look forward to. But Dr. Rosen's words were far better than a party. However, they also emphasized the danger of 5-FU and the severity of its side effects. I was suddenly proud of myself for making it as far as I did.

"So, what's next?" I asked.

"We will monitor your health each year for the next five years."

"How will you do that?" Debbie asked.

Although Debbie asked the question, Dr. Rosen's eyes remained fixed on mine. "We'll give you a few months off, and then we'll do a CT scan of your chest, abdomen, and the pelvis, which will include the liver. We'll also do the usual blood tests and consultation and follow that with a colonoscopy."

"How about the side effects I'm experiencing?" I asked.

"With time they should ease," she said. "And any hair you lost should grow back. The only thing that could remain is the neuropathy in your fingers and feet. This part of the recovery is different for each person."

The part about the hair was good news. I had only lost about one third of my hair, and that was mostly thinning. Each time I showered I lost small amounts, so I didn't know what it was like to be temporarily bald. But I didn't like her answer about the neuropathy. "How long will it be until I'll know?"

"I can't answer that," she replied. "I know cases where feeling has returned immediately, but then others just learn to live with it."

I nodded as if I understood, but it was another unknown I had to face. I certainly hoped I was one of the lucky ones who regained feeling. Then I touched the bump under my shirt and asked, "What about the Portacath? When do I get it out?"

Dr. Rosen was quick and confident with her reply. "Most of my patients choose to leave it in. I advise you to do the same."

The thought of living with the Portacath inside my body when it really didn't need to be there was as nauseating as if I were actually having a chemotherapy treatment. "Why do most of your patients choose to leave it in?"

Dr. Rosen answered with a question. "Why not?" She paused and slightly cocked her head. Her expression revealed her authority and the fact that she had dealt with the question on many occasions. When I didn't reply she continued, "It's not causing you any harm, and there's always the chance that you might need it again. Of course, we would need to flush the port with a saline solution once a month."

I tried to ignore what she inferred, but the message was loud and clear. I knew she was right. We went into this treatment with a positive attitude and hope, but we also knew there were no guarantees. I was not a quitter, but I didn't know if I could handle a repeat performance. How many times could I have cancer and endure chemotherapy? And how many times could I win the battle?

Suddenly, I felt Debbie's hand on my knee. I knew from her touch that she understood the anguish I was experiencing. "Maybe we need time to think about it a little longer," she said, looking up at Dr. Rosen.

Dr. Rosen nodded.

"No!" I exclaimed. I was as shocked as Debbie and Dr. Rosen at my tone. "I've already made my decision. I want it out."

Dr. Rosen shot me her I'm-the-physician look. "Maybe we should wait a few weeks as your wife suggested, Mr. Yates."

"I don't need to wait," I said calmer. "My decision is final."

Dr. Rosen was annoyed. "Have you given any thought as to what happens if your cancer does return? You'll have to have another port inserted."

"Don't you see?" I asked. "If I leave the Portacath in, I'll constantly be reminded of the possibility of a reoccurrence. It'll be as though the cancer has a hold on my life, like it controls me, just waiting for the opportunity to rob me of my life again. I don't want to live like that. Removing it is a positive statement that I am not going to be a prisoner to cancer. My mind is made up. I want it out."

To my surprise, as irritated as Dr. Rosen had been only moments before, she now appeared as if nothing had happened. "Very well," she said. "It's your decision. But I do caution you, Mr. Yates, that if the cancer does return, we have to act fast."

I held firm. "I understand. If and when that time comes, I'll be ready and will follow your advice unquestionably. But at this time, I want it out, and I'm going to schedule an appointment with Dr. Sparrow."

She shook Debbie's hand and then mine. "My coordinator will be in touch with you in a few months to schedule your first checkup." She actually developed a half smile. "Congratulations on making it this far."

Debbie and I left Dr. Rosen's office at ten thirty. Silence prevailed much of the ride home. As we drove, I had one thing on my mind—magic mushrooms. I didn't know what to expect, but at eleven o'clock I took my first dose of the supplement. I was thinking it might immediately make me strong, like Popeye after eating a can of spinach, but nothing happened. Was I really so foolish as to think that one dose would take away my cancer and restore me to the person I used to be? Perhaps the thought had been hovering subconsciously all this time, but, regardless, I was determined to stay the course. From the Japanese studies, I knew they worked. I was prepared to take them faithfully in the dosage recommended on the label— one to three capsules twice daily on an empty stomach. I had already mentally made them part of my daily regime and part of who I was.

My eyes drifted to the spice cabinet where the 5-FU pills were stashed, and a force drew me to them like a magnetic field. My hand was shaking as I grabbed the bottle and ran to the bathroom, and then I dumped the poison pills into the toilet. I flushed it twice to make sure they were all gone. Either there were going to be a lot of cancer-free sewer rats or a ton of dead ones. Relief washed over me. I felt free.

By Friday I was feeling better than I had in months. I don't know if it was the monthly B-12 shot I had on Thursday, the magic mushrooms, or the mental relief that I was through with chemotherapy—or a combination of all three. It could have been my scheduled surgical appointment the following week to have Dr. Sparrow remove the Portacath—the procedure was quick and successful and I was in and out of the same-day surgical clinic at University Hospital in four hours. Whatever the reason, I was feeling normal again.

The following months ticked away slowly, as did my recovery. The nausea had subsided, although at least once a week I suffered from a chemo day, a condition most of the medical profession refuses to acknowledge. Whether it is psychological or physical, it makes no difference. The fact remains that it happens and I never know when it is going to occur. At least during chemotherapy I knew when and how long to expect the sickness.

My cognitive skills got better, but I have yet to return to what I call normal. Especially during a chemo day, a foggy cloud hangs over me. I usually spend this time either resting on the couch or watching a ballgame on television, anything to help me keep my mind away from the porcelain god. Or I go for walks around the park with Debbie. And during this time, I don't dare try to multitask.

I religiously continued the magic mushrooms—I was elated to find new information on the Internet about new studies and actual clinical trials being conducted by some physicians in the United States, which made me all the more determined to continue the supplement—and upgraded my exercise. I worked out at our community gym three times a week and walked daily with Debbie. And although my strength increased weekly, most of my side effects still existed. I realized it was going to be a long road with lots of obstacles, but I was never going to quit. I had promised Mary.

CHAPTER 18

Camp Keepsake

MID-JUNE of 2007, Debbie saw an article in the newspaper advertising a camp for cancer survivors. Immediately she thought of our situation and knew it was a great idea, but my initial reaction was cold. "Those camps and discussions are not for me," I protested stiffly. "The last thing I want to do is sit around and talk about cancer and chemotherapy with people I don't even know."

As was now the norm in our lives, Debbie wanted me to continue to do everything on my end to make sure I survived cancer, and she considered this to be part of my recovery. She strongly encouraged me—which included a little nagging. "It's for the entire family," she explained. "Amanda and I can both attend with you. I think we all might benefit from it."

Against my better judgment, I downloaded an application for Camp Keepsake from the Cancer Hope Foundation Web site whose headquarters were only about ten miles south of Santa Domingo.

I filled out the application, but part of the needed information had to be supplied by a physician. I called Dr. Rosen's office and talked to her coordinator. She said I was on her list to call for my first checkup and CT scan, so we scheduled it for July 10. I decided to wait until then to take the forms to Dr. Rosen. The final date for applying to the camp was July 31, well over a month away.

The more I thought about it, the more I realized I definitely didn't want to participate in a camp for cancer survivors. It sounded like a dumb idea, like swapping stories about Vietnam with a bunch of complaining veterans. However, I was merely applying to the camp. It certainly didn't mean that I would be accepted. Chances were, so many applicants would be ahead of me that my application would be pushed far under the stack...I hoped.

On Tuesday, July 10, I met with Dr. Rosen in her office. She agreed to fill out the physician's section of the application and fax it to the Cancer Hope Foundation. As far as I was concerned, that was the end of it, although she did agree with Debbie that it might be a beneficial experience.

My blood panel revealed that all categories were in the good range, especially the red and white blood cell counts. We discussed the remaining side effects I still experienced: chemo days about once a week, chronic fatigue, neuropathy in my fingers and toes, and itching and flushing face (my cognitive impairments were still my secret). My taste buds appeared to have returned from their sabbatical over the past couple of weeks, and the woman who cuts my hair informed me that black hair was growing in the thinnest area over the top of my head. That was good news, though I'd never had black hair before.

Dr. Rosen didn't appear concerned about any of the side effects. She scheduled me for a CT scan. A week and a half later, I was back in her office with the results.

"After reviewing these reports, Mr. Yates, you appear to be doing quite well. Your lungs are clear, and there is no evidence of cancer in your liver or pelvic area. There is, however, a small dark spot on the liver, but it appears to be just that, a dark spot."

And that was it. She scheduled an appointment for a colonoscopy with a physician in the same building. So far, as she saw it, my recovery was going well.

I was also extremely happy with the checkup, and even more excited to share the information with Debbie, but I couldn't figure out why Dr. Rosen wasn't concerned by the side effects I still experienced from the chemotherapy. Debbie reasoned that, from the physician's point of view, they were happy when patients survived, at least temporarily—side effects were trivial compared to living. This rationalization actually made sense, but in no way did it diminish the daily discomfort I experienced. I will admit that the longer I live and enjoy life, the easier it is to cope, and I will never abandon hope that one day I will be free from all of the side effects.

I received a letter in the mail on August 15 from the Cancer Hope Foundation. My family and I had been selected to attend Camp Keepsake.

I should have been elated, jumping with joy, but instead, I was already trying to figure a way out of it. Debbie came into the kitchen before I could slide the letter to the bottom of the stack of bills and advertisements.

"What's that?"

I've never been able to bluff Debbie. She can read my thoughts as if they were displayed on my forehead, especially if I attempt to bend the truth. I was trapped, so I said, "A letter from the Cancer Hope Foundation about that camp you were interested in."

Debbie grabbed the letter and read that we'd been accepted. "This is great news," she said joyfully.

"Maybe," I reluctantly replied, "but I don't know if I want to go."

"I thought we agreed to give it a try if we were given the opportunity."

"I just said that because I didn't think we would be accepted."

I hadn't seen "the look" in quite some time; in fact, I've rarely seen it from Debbie in twenty years of marriage, but there it was. There was nothing I could say or do to get out of the situation, so I uttered a low, "I'm sorry."

"The look" softened.

"Please give it a try," she said. "You might be surprised and enjoy it."

"How can sitting around with a bunch of people I don't know talking about everyone's experience with cancer and maybe singing 'Kumbaya' be enjoyable? It's hard enough talking about it with people I know."

Debbie was quick to remind me that we had looked at the camp's Web site. "There's more to it than that, and you know it."

A long moment elapsed before I reluctantly agreed. "Okay, I'll give it a try." I said it, but I didn't mean it. The camp was a month and a half away, and with a little luck, something more pressing in our lives would intervene.

Camp Keepsake is a unique program unlike any I have ever seen or heard of. An incredible nonprofit organization, Cancer Hope Foundation, started this camp for adults with cancer, those undergoing chemotherapy, those in remission, and those who are considered survivors. Depending on the number of slots available, the camp allows up to five family members and/or friends to attend with the applicant.

Camp Keepsake is located in a wilderness setting in the coastal mountains of Malibu and is much more than a camp for talking about cancer experiences. There are numerous games, activities, music, dancing, and they even have a spa for massages, facials, and pedicures. And the camp is totally free for all applicants and family members.

There is the opportunity to share your experiences with cancer if you so desire, but there is never any pressure. I laughed, cried, and learned many valuable lessons of caring, kindness, and compassion that have helped my spirit grow. Camp Keepsake motivated me to write this book.

There was no earth-shattering event or family crisis that developed over the next month, so on Friday, October 5, at four thirty in the afternoon, Debbie, Amanda, and I drove through the entrance to Camp Keepsake. We found ourselves in orderly chaos amid campers, staff, and volunteers, not to mention a two-piece band off to our left playing songs from the early sixties.

There were several cars in line ahead of us, so we waited for the next available volunteer, a curly-haired woman in her fifties, "Lois" was on her nametag, and on her face was the smile of an angel. She welcomed us just as two more vibrant volunteers arrived in a golf cart and unloaded our bags.

We were treated with more respect and love than dignitaries, but the wall of caution I had built while in Vietnam remained intact. There was a catch somewhere—there had to be—because no one displayed this level of kindness without a motive. The only exceptions in my life had been my mother, Debbie, Mary, and my chemotherapy nurses.

We checked in and received a schedule for the next three days, and each of us was given a white camp T-shirt in our size. It read, "Camp Keepsake, European Connection, 2007."

As we left the check-in booth, mesmerized by the buzz of energetic campers, we met our host for the weekend, a handsome young volunteer named Jake, who was in his late twenties, well built, and a couple of inches taller than me. He was soft spoken and sincere, that much I could tell. Debbie and Amanda instantly adopted him and gave him a big hug, though I only shook his hand. My wall was still my protection.

Jake showed us to our dormitory-style rooms so we could get settled and then met us at what I'll call the mess hall—a centrally located building that housed a commercial kitchen and dining area, bathrooms, and a huge gathering room with a stone fireplace and a piano. The room was arranged with twenty large circular tables and chairs for eating.

We listened to welcome speeches as we ate, enjoying chicken Marsala, salad, bread, and dessert that left me stuffed. Jake was with us the entire time and introduced us to staff, volunteers, and other campers. I saw men, women, and kids of all ages and nationalities and religion as well. Some looked as healthy as I did, and some wore bandanas or hats on bald heads. Others sat in wheelchairs or used walkers. I also noticed that everyone in the building had something in common other than cancer: they appeared to be enjoying themselves—their smiles were triumphant. Cancer may have claimed parts of their lives, but at the moment, "Survivors ruled and cancer drooled."

We were free for forty-five minutes and chose to scout the valley that held this magnificent camp. There were four barrack-style buildings near the entrance with centrally located baths and showers in each, a large octagonal entertainment and meeting building, the mess hall, a building designated as a sick bay, and a three-story hotel-style structure where all of the amenities for the weekend were offered. There was a large grassy area in the center of camp for sports, crafts, and activities; a small outdoor stage with benches for bands and dancing; and there was a miniature amphitheater with concrete bench seating and a centrally located fire pit.

At seven o'clock most of the campers and their families flocked to the amphitheater for something I found very moving: a drum circle. We came upon drums—hundreds of drums—bongos and Native American tom-toms of all sizes and shapes to drum sticks, cowbells, and tambourines.

Debbie, Amanda, and I each picked up a drum and met Jake near the top of the theater. And then we drummed.

There was a leader in the center by the fire pit who directed the tribe of drummers unlike anything I had ever seen. No matter what or how each person played, he somehow managed to arrange the beating into a symphony.

I played continually for an hour, sometimes loud, then soft, and then there were times I just banged as if I wanted to destroy the drum. It suddenly represented all of the bad things that had happened in my life. I pounded it for my mother, for others I had known who had suffered from cancer, for my own cancers, for everyone and their families in the amphitheater who were waging battles of their own every day. And I pounded for Mary. Then, the drumming took on an unbelievable pulse of its own, like a strong heartbeat. It was as if everyone in the amphitheatre had come together as one, resulting in the rhythmic beating of one colossal heart.

As I thought of Mary, tears rolled from my eyes onto the drum. Then I drummed with more vigor. There wasn't a day that I didn't think of her. I knew she was spiritually with me, but I wanted her to be physically here now.

She would love this place and everyone would have loved her, but all I could do for her was beat a drum.

We finished drumming at eight o'clock, and as soon as Debbie heard the band playing Beatles' songs, we were off to the outdoor stage. Jake came with us and danced with Amanda and Debbie and a number of others. I sat on a bench mesmerized by the spirit and electricity radiating from everyone I observed. It seemed as though all inhibitions had been abandoned, except for mine. But that only lasted a short time, as Jake, Debbie, Amanda, and what seemed like everyone we had already met, coaxed me to the dance floor.

Suddenly, I felt as if I had known these people all of my life. Before I could talk myself out of it, I dropped my wall, but not completely. I danced, laughed, and had fun without caring what people thought. And the best part was the smile on Debbie's face; it was one I'll never forget—and one that reminded me of how much she loved me.

We danced and sang along with the band until ten. I was exhausted, but I couldn't remember the last time I'd had so much fun.

Debbie, Amanda, and Jake, along with a host of others, wanted coffee and s'mores around the fire pit in the amphitheater, so I said good night to a group of wonderful people I had not known six hours earlier and headed for the dormitory room.

I remember nothing else that night, except my head hitting the pillow, but I'm sure I had a smile on my face that reflected the past six hours of my life. Little did I know that the smiles and laughter had only just begun.

Saturday morning, Debbie and I were up early. We took an hour-long hike before breakfast with a dozen other early risers along a nature trail in the surrounding mountains. The air was amazingly fresh and crisp; it rejuvenated our lungs and I felt lucky to be alive.

After breakfast, Debbie and Amanda had pre-arranged times for facials, pedicures, and massages. Though I'm not a fan of spa treatments, I did have a massage, which was actually very enjoyable.

Throughout the day there were games and crafts, including a climbing wall and a reptilian exhibit. I wasn't into the games and crafts, although I did make a tie-dye shirt with Amanda—purple and gold for LSU.

One of the best things about Camp Keepsake and its personnel is that nothing is expected of the campers. Each person participates in events as much or little as desired. There is absolutely no pressure.

Dinner was another delicious meal of chicken, tri-tip, veggies, salad, and cake for dessert. We sat at a table with Jake and five other women we had not met. Two of the women, with whom I chatted most of the time, were cancer and chemotherapy survivors. They told me about the continuing side effects of their treatments.

Though their cancers were different than mine, as were their chemotherapy treatments, they still had many of the side effects that affected me. And the emotional uncertainty and pain was still there. One petite woman of about fifty-five had survived breast cancer for five years. The other, a fifty-nine-year-old plump woman with shoulder-length gray hair, had survived lung cancer for three years.

As with my symptoms, their biggest complaint was fatigue and nausea during an occasional chemo day. Neither one had experienced neuropathy of the fingers or toes, but a woman with whom I talked later, who had surgery for 2-A colon cancer, still experienced neuropathy, fatigue, chemo days, and flushness in her face; she had been off chemo for almost four years.

While I was grateful for the information they shared, it was disappointing to realize that I could possibly have side effects for years to come. I had been off chemotherapy for nine months, and although I knew chemicals affected people differently, I was secretly praying that I didn't have to go through the side effects described by my two new friends for five more years.

At least I learned that my symptoms were real and not a figment of my imagination, as most of those in the medical profession inferred. It was actually comforting to be validated.

Earlier in the day, all campers and family members had been given a blank scroll and asked to write their thoughts about cancer, life, or family-related issues—whatever came from their hearts.

At seven o'clock, we gathered at the amphitheater for the "Wishful Scroll Ceremony." Jake, the other campers and their families, hosts, volunteers, and the staff of the Cancer Hope Foundation were all there. It was a Camp Keepsake tradition that each family got a turn on the small stage in front of the circular fire pit to say a few words about their camp experience, cancer, the staff, or whatever touched them. Or they could say nothing at all and just toss the scroll into the fire. The camp's position was that no matter what was written on the scroll (i.e., "cancer sucks") would be burned and the ashes mixed with the ashes of all the scrolls burned over the past seven years at Camp Keepsake. It was a way to connect everyone with their trials, tribulations, and successes; more importantly, it was a gesture of the unity of our souls crying out with a passion to defeat this intruder in our lives.

I found the ceremony very emotional and spiritually poignant. At times it had a touch of humor, much sadness, and quite a bit of triumph.

The ceremony began alphabetically, so, naturally, we were going to be near the end, if not last. We listened to stories of remission and survival, tragic stories of reoccurrence, stories of beautiful people and friends taking care of loved ones undergoing chemotherapy. There were several stories of people who had no more fight left in them. They were tired and felt that it was their time to let go. This nearly broke my heart, and I immediately thought of Mary uttering the same words. In my mind I yelled, "Never give up! Never ever give up!"

The ceremony lasted an hour and a half. Every emotion I had ever experienced surfaced and claimed my thoughts. It was almost as if my entire life played before me as I listened to the real drama on the stage below: Vietnam, with the horrors and torture of a country in turmoil and the disregard for human life on both sides; my earlier battles with malignant melanoma and the change it made in my life; my mother's suffering and death from lung and bone cancer and my understanding of why and how something good can result from a tragic event or death; and, of course, my recent battle with an old nemesis: cancer.

At the end of each short speech there were applause as a member of each family tossed the scroll into the fire. As small or large as it was, it was a moment of personal triumph for each family. And the crowd acknowledged their special moment.

And then I heard, "David Yates and family."

We made our way down the steps to the stage and stood at the microphone before what seemed like a thousand people. Jake was with us. The little rehearsal I had done a hundred times over the past couple of hours escaped me as if I had amnesia, but I could never forget why I was here. So I winged it.

I introduced Debbie, Amanda, and Jake before I said, "This is an incredible place." A section of the crowd cheered, probably not because of what I said, but most likely because they knew I was the last one to speak.

"This has certainly been a humbling experience, one I will never forget. From the moment we arrived, my family and I have been treated like royalty, and the atmosphere here is what everyone dreams for and hopes will happen to our world: compassion and equality. Thank you to the Cancer Hope Foundation, all of the volunteers, and especially to Jake, our host. Thank you for having Debbie, Amanda, and me. Just as with every one of you, what is written on this scroll is from our hearts, and my wish is that, for everyone here, it will come true. Thank you."

Debbie and I chose Amanda to toss the scroll into the fire. There were more cheers, the Master of Ceremonies thanked everyone, and then it was over.

As I stood watching everyone leave, confusion coursed through me. I felt rejuvenated, as if a thousand-pound weight had been lifted from me. I felt whole and pure like the first snowflake of winter and as strong as a gale-force wind. Yet I was saddened by the thought of this being over. I would probably never see these people again. And how many would soon lose their battles?

Sleep escaped me most of the night, but when I did slip into the realm of self-awareness, I saw the entire camp as a unified, triumphant whole, celebrating the victory over cancer. But I also saw a small group hovering overhead, those who would not make it much longer. This was disheartening, but I again found mystical solace within the large group.

The following morning, I wasn't the same person I had been the day before. My mood was somber, yet I did my best to smile and laugh with every camper and staff person I encountered. I could tell there were others who felt the same way, yet they, too, masked their feelings.

After breakfast we all met in the large octagonal building near the barracks to see a slide show of the hundreds of pictures taken over the past two days. There were smiles, laughter, tears, and a lot of hugs. And then, the camp I had so desperately tried to avoid was over. Worse, my wall had returned.

Volunteers brought all of our gear from the barracks as we stood by the curb with our host waiting for our car to be delivered to us. Different volunteers loaded the car as we said our good-byes to Jake. Debbie and Amanda were first, and then my handshake with Jake turned into an enormous bear hug. As we separated, tears glistened in both of our eyes.

"Thanks," I said, "for making us feel so welcome and special. I'll never forget you."

Jake only nodded, because I don't think he could get words past the lump that had grown in his throat, the same lump I was experiencing. I'll always remember the love and kindness he showed us, as did every other volunteer and staff person, but most of all, I will remember what he said the day before, when we talked about Mary.

"You're fortunate to have had someone like her in your life. A lot of people who undergo chemotherapy and/or radiation have no Mary, and many don't have the support of family or friends. You're a stronger person from knowing her, and it's your turn to be there for someone else."

Who was this young man with such wisdom?

To this day I am convinced that he was yet another who was destined to be in my life during one of my life challenges. If we are judged by what we do for others and how we make them feel, then Jake is not only an incredible human being but will be at the top of the list in the Kingdom of God .

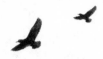

CHAPTER 19

Meditation

SOME YEARS ago I learned to meditate. It had nothing to do with religion, yet the actual experience was extremely spiritual, allowing me to travel deep within my soul in search of relief from anxiety and stress. It became a place to look for answers to any and all questions that have ever entered my thoughts.

Not only was meditation (referred to by some as hypnosis, yoga, or even prayer) a spiritual experience, but it also made me a better person, especially in the kindness and compassion department. For some reason, during the year in which I battled colon cancer, I had stopped this personal ritual, but during Camp Keepsake I scheduled an appointment with a hypnotist. Though I wasn't actually hypnotized, I experienced a very relaxed state and my previous meditation techniques resurfaced.

Perhaps this experience is not for everyone, as we all have our own beliefs, likes, and dislikes, but there may be some who find it useful. Here's what I do.

I begin by lying flat on my back in a comfortable position with my arms at my sides, or I sit in the traditional yoga position, *sukhasana*, with my back straight, the backs of my hands resting on my knees with my palms up, and my thumbs and index fingers touching. I suggest experimenting to find whatever variation of either method is best for you. The most important ingredients I have found are to be in a comfortable, relaxed position and a noise- and interference-free environment.

With my eyes closed, I breathe deeply and expel the air slowly as many times as it takes until my body feels light and my mind grows unaware of my physical surroundings. It's almost like a kneading cat that finally finds the perfect spot.

When I'm ready, I focus on a stairway, one I remember as a teen. The stairway is wide and has an oak railing and wooden steps with blue carpet runners down the middle. It can be whatever you want it to be—wide, narrow, spiral, elegant, or as rustic as a cabin. There are no rules except to relax, to focus on letting go of a particular problem, or to achieve the answer to a question.

I visualize myself slowly descending the steps, one at a time while counting from ten to one, and with each step, I release stress and anxiety until I experience extreme serenity at the end.

When I lower myself from the last step, I'm always with my mother, something I plan before my journey. Whether I meet her in her kitchen frying chicken or in church singing one of the old hymns she loved, I always choose a soul-enriching memory. She is my guide, my comforter, the center of happy times as a child, and my earthly example of love and kindness. We hug and talk for a moment before she leads me to a door, the reason I have come.

I open the door and step over the threshold to find myself standing at the pinnacle of a mountain, one of the many tranquil places I choose during such encounters. (Again, it can be any place that brings you comfort.) I stand looking over a luscious green valley with a river meandering through it.

I see a bright light in the distance that moves toward me and suddenly is upon me and engulfs me. The light is brilliant, yet soft and easy on my eyes.

I am not afraid; rather, I'm as peaceful as a nursing child. The energy from the light radiates through me and I feel kindness, compassion, and love. The knowledge of forgiveness is overpowering. My thoughts as to why I am here are openly revealed. Soon the answers I have sought are known or the anxiety I have felt is released.

I stand basking in the warmth and understanding until I realize the light has left. I feel as if the light still engulfs me. At this point, although I have no understanding of how much time has passed, I know I must return.

I step back over the threshold and close the door. My mother is still frying chicken. The aroma is as mouthwatering as it was when I was a child. She has her back to me and is singing an old hymn. I hug her and tell her I love her, but she already knows this. I don't want to leave, but I must, for to remain in this state would take me away from Debbie and the physical world I still love. I walk to the stairway and put my foot on the first step. I turn, and she is no longer there.

I slowly ascend the stairs, and with each step I retain the peacefulness left by my journey. When I reach the top step, I open my eyes. I am always smiling and I feel a deep sense of love.

How much time has elapsed is always different. I have spent as little as fifteen minutes on one of these journeys and as long as an hour and a half on what I am seeking. But regardless of the time, I have always returned with answered questions and renewed love and forgiveness for those I encounter in everyday life.

How often do I do this? Usually once a day, sometimes twice. My favorite time to meditate is early morning before a new day begins, but if the opportunity presents itself, I am ready. This daily practice helps me to keep my wall down.

So, with all of this kindness, compassion, love, and forgiveness I must be the perfect man, right? Not even close. I am still a physical being on this earth with a spiritual awareness that distinguishes who I am. I still get disappointed, feisty, and even angry, but the God within me soon prevails.

Do I have to do this every day? I don't think so, but it is something I look forward to. It has become a part of my total being, much the same as eating and breathing.

There are those who would call what I do heretical and blasphemous, yet I am not involving any religion. I am simply learning what life is about and why I am here. I am learning to be more tolerant of all human beings regardless of race, religion, or gender. And I am learning love and forgiveness as I believe my creator intended.

CHAPTER 20

Camp Keepsake 2 and 3

FOUR YEARS have passed since my last chemotherapy treatment and I am still plagued with some of the side effects: fatigue, an occasional chemo day, flushed face, neuropathy in my feet, and a light-headedness that refuses to leave, much like a house guest who has overstayed his welcome.

Each year I've had a CT scan of my liver and chest, a colonoscopy, and blood tests. With each test, the results have been positive. Only the colonoscopy revealed any anomaly. One new polyp had formed each year and was removed.

The gastrointestinal staff initially refused my request for a colonoscopy each year. At first I couldn't believe they would turn away business, but their justification was that the insurance company would not approve another one so soon. However, Dr. Rosen and I were unrelenting. The insurance company did approve the procedure, and now I was elated that I had an oncologist and/or hematologist who was aggressive and took charge. Not only do I think she is a good physician, I actually like her. She is definitely Glinda, the good and caring witch.

The will to live is a very powerful force. Sometimes we cannot take no for an answer. If we do not fight for ourselves, who is going to?

Physicians are mortal men and women just like all of us. Yes, they are educated and trained in healing and/or relieving pain, but they are not gods. We are our best physicians and we must rely on ourselves and demand proper care. To do so is to join the fight to eliminate cancer.

Debbie, Amanda, and I have attended Camp Keepsake three years in a row, and each camp has been better than its predecessor. It's not because the camp had better food or activities, but because I was more open and receptive to the kindness, compassion, and love of the staff, volunteers, and campers.

My second Camp Keepsake was wonderful. Under pressure from Debbie, I agreed to have a pedicure; as unmanly as it may seem to some, it was more stimulating than a full-body massage. I think the manicurist who performed the delicate treatment was as excited to perform on a "pedicure virgin" as I was to have it.

My wall, which had been up for much of the previous year, took a beating from the moment we arrived. By Saturday evening at the Wishful Scroll Ceremony it had crumbled like the Berlin Wall. But it wasn't just the normal kindness, compassion, and love that kept my wall down most of the following year, it was a special young woman.

I had seen her throughout the weekend but did not talk to her. She was tall and thin and wore a skin-tone bandage covering the left side of her face from just below her eyebrow to the middle of her cheek. She was in her early forties and seemed to be enjoying the special atmosphere.

I had never heard of cancer of the eye, but I was rapidly learning that cancer did not discriminate when it came to which part of the body it chose to infiltrate.

Everyone who spoke that night touched my heart with a comment or story of tragedy or victory, but this special woman reached my soul. She spoke briefly about losing her eye to cancer, but the powerful message she gave about Camp Keepsake was what arrested my attention. She described it as the only place she had been since her fight began where she felt as though she blended in. She felt safe and knew people were not staring at her as if she were a circus freak. I knew exactly what she meant. To say I was moved would never give justice to the power of what she said.

Since my first cancer surgery in 1969, I have always worn clothes that conceal the scars on my neck. I felt as though I wasn't complete and that people looked at me as less of a person. But that night at the Wishful Scroll Ceremony changed everything for me. From the moment I heard her words, I was no longer ashamed of my scarred body. I decided that I was as physically perfect as I needed to be, and I would no longer allow anyone to look down on me. I was a spirit, and spiritual rules. I was going to present myself with confidence as an equal member of society.

It was also the moment I realized why I had built such a massive wall and kept it raised since Vietnam. That night was the beginning of a different way of life for me— one without a wall.

My third Camp Keepsake was again a weekend of paradise on earth. I had managed to keep my wall down during most of the year, yet a few months earlier I allowed a stressful situation to temporarily control my life. The wall had surfaced. However, it immediately came down as soon as we drove into the camp and were greeted by kindness, compassion, and love that would follow us the entire weekend. Our host, Sara, was a friend from past years who epitomized the goal of Camp Keepsake in all aspects of her life.

Once again, I was moved by some of the stories that campers and staff shared at the Wishful Scroll Ceremony. Most were heartbreaking, yet triumphant. The survivors would most likely be around for another Camp Keepsake, but, as always, there were a few who revealed that perhaps the end of the journey was near for them.

For me, the camp allowed me to drop my wall and take risks, encouraged by the staff and volunteers. I love attending this camp, and the people I've befriended are all courageous and loving. Every time I'm with them, their kindness and compassion reminds me of Mary, and she is someone I never want to forget.

If I were the most valuable player of the Super Bowl and was asked the familiar question, "Now that you've won the big game, what are you going to do next?" my answer would be, "I'm going to Camp Keepsake." For me and many others it is truly the *Magic Kingdom*.

Thanks to the Cancer Hope Foundation's staff, hosts, and volunteers for making a lot of dreams come true. You really do make a huge difference in all of our lives.

As I write this, cancer continues to wreck the lives of those around me. A former coworker is fighting prostate cancer, a woman is receiving treatment for cancer of the nose, a neighbor is still fighting after eighteen years of cancer and remission, and an elderly man's body is so riddled with cancer that he will lose his battle within the month. A friend has just lost both breasts to cancer, and another friend—after surviving throat cancer for three years—is recovering from chemotherapy and radiation for lung cancer.

There appears to be no end. One in six of those I mentioned will die within the month (I actually just learned that the elderly man has given up his fight). One or two of the others will most likely lose their battle before the five-year mark. But the remaining three will beat the odds—a better percentage than five years ago. And the next five years will yield an even higher survival percentage, as will the next, and the next, until there is an end.

How do I know there will be an end to cancer? I hear it with every breath I take. I feel it with every normal cell in my body, and I see it in every cancer sufferer who refuses to quit. We all have within us that God-given will to live and enjoy the world around us, but that alone is sometimes not enough to continue individual battles. I hope that each one who reads this will reach out and be there for another who is fighting alone. It can and will make a huge difference in our struggle to be cancer free.

EPILOGUE

CANCER SUCKS!

LIKE EVERYONE on this earth, I have faced a number of life challenges. But I have also had my share of life pleasures. How is it possible to know one without the other? For me, surviving cancer is definitely a life pleasure.

It has been thirty years since my mother's death due to cancer, and it's taken me this long to understand what she meant by, "No matter what happens in your life, there is always the opportunity to take good from it." All of these years I've wondered how there could be good from her death, but, like a life pleasure, it can be anything we want it to be. The good is left for each of us to discover.

Many of the simple things in life I've always taken for granted now have new meaning: Walking barefoot in a field of grass, watching a colorful sunset, feeling the rough bark of an oak tree, and smelling the thick fragrance of a rose in full bloom. A deep breath on a crisp fall morning is something I will always long for, and the sweetness of a fresh summer pear will forever remain etched in my mind.

Perhaps I will never know what really caused my bout with malignant melanoma in 1968 (although I am convinced it was caused by Agent Orange), but what I do know is that there are many things I could have done to combat the disease. I should have avoided direct sun as much as possible, especially because I am fair-skinned and subject to quick burning, and I should have used plenty of sunscreen during exposure. But as a teenager living in South Florida, sunscreen wasn't a cool thing to do, and it wasn't part of the Army's standard equipment issue. Unfortunately, most of today's teens love tanning booths and direct sun.

I now know not to wear jewelry such as necklaces, bracelets, watches, and rings that constantly rub or irritate a mole or any area of skin that could be susceptible to developing cancer. The dog tags I had to wear around my neck during the war in Vietnam could have been the reason for cancer (although most dermatologists believe emphatically that melanoma can only be caused by overexposure to ultraviolet rays). And I also now know what to look for when I do a daily inspection of my body. Awareness can actually save your life.

I have also learned to avoid chemicals and pesticides as often as I can, but today's world is full of poisonous cleaning products that are difficult to avoid, just as it is difficult to avoid the fallout from agricultural spraying. I even wear rubber gloves for household chores that require chemical cleaners and disinfectants. I suggest that everyone wear them.

As for colon cancer, it is widely encouraged to have a colonoscopy at age fifty, or earlier, if there is a family history of cancer. Do not wait for your primary care physician (PCP) to recommend one. Be proactive and demand the procedure. If your PCP will not give you a referral, find another provider. A colonoscopy is literally as easy as passing gas. We know our own bodies, and we must never allow physicians or our government to make final decisions concerning our health.

If you are diagnosed with colon cancer, fight it. Was I afraid of the unknown? Yes. But when I decided to do everything I could to rid myself of this dreaded disease, I found I had strength I didn't know I possessed.

If surgery is necessary, remember that we all have our choice of surgeons. Find one who has a good reputation for the actual surgery, but also a person in whom you have confidence and who will take the time to answer questions and provide answers. I had confidence in my PCP and used the surgeon he recommended. However, the final decision was mine. And check on the latest advances in surgical procedures, including robotic surgery.

If I were faced with another surgery, I would use pain medication only when necessary (austerity could prevent hallucinations and addiction problems). And after the surgery, I would also walk as much and as often as I could, because exercise is an important part of remaining healthy.

A blockage is certainly possible while recovering from surgery. I strongly recommend following the physician's instructions for a soft diet, and if I had to face recovery again, I would extend the time by another week or two, slowly introducing my body to easily digestible solid food. And remember, chew your food thoroughly.

If chemotherapy is recommended, make sure the hematologist/oncologist is established and aware of the latest methods and available medicines, and do your own homework. Research everything you can about the chemicals to be used and the possible side effects to your body. I liked the fact that Dr. Rosen was aggressive and spent as much time with me as I needed during office visits, though she did not have all of the answers to my questions. But never forget that the final decision is left to each of us. I would also suggest checking out the nurses who will be administering your cocktail. Spend at least half an hour in the treatment room observing their interactions with other patients. It's an extremely important part of the puzzle when undergoing chemotherapy.

Surgery for a Portacath is another unknown that can be frightening, but it takes about the same length of time as a colonoscopy and is just as easy—only three to four hours in same-day surgery. For the number of punctures required for lengthy chemotherapy, this is the way to go. There is a short recovery time after the surgery, a lump under your skin that is often an emotional reminder of what is happening in your life on a daily basis, and there will be a small scar.

As I said earlier, the horrors of Vietnam weren't as frightening as the unknown of the first day of chemotherapy. It was overwhelming, but, for me, it was my own imagination that caused my grief. As anxious as I was, I knew to ask Dr. Rosen for something to calm me. She agreed and ordered Ativan. It also helped, at least during the first treatment, to have someone with me; a spouse or friend can make a huge difference in your level of anxiety. And remember, the monster I expected never surfaced.

The Oxaliplatin was easy—I had no discomfort or sickness. The 5-FU doesn't hurt and you don't feel it (and I did get used to the *click-clunk* of the pump after the first night), but there most likely will be side effects. And remember, I believe the iPod and headphones helped with my anxiety and nausea.

I've learned that the side effects are definitely different with each person, yet the most common ones shared by most chemotherapy patients are nausea and fatigue.

I still experience some side effects, which remain a part of my life four years after my last chemotherapy treatment.

I still have chemo days once or twice a month. It's something I think we all just learn to live with. The nausea will not completely leave me, but I experience it less with each passing year.

Fatigue is simply part of my life. I have not returned to the level of energy I used to possess, but I feel pretty good most days. I experience three to four days of extreme fatigue every month—even without a chemo day. On these days it is hard to even get out of bed. But I've learned that if I don't give in to the demands and remain active (especially walking and exercising), I can usually overcome the exhaustion.

My problem with cognitive functioning was quite real. Please do not let anyone tell you "It's nothing associated with the chemicals," or "You're just getting older and this is how aging works," or "It's just in your head." Of course it's in our heads. Some physicians don't like being faced with questions to which they have no answers, so they offer a statement like, "I've found nothing in your tests that would indicate a connection between chemotherapy and the cognitive impairments you are suggesting." Be prepared to have lots of questions with few answers, but remember that most of the cognitive issues should subside after chemotherapy is finished.

I was hit with confusion, concentration issues, short-term memory loss, and problems with multitasking, especially during the first week of chemotherapy. For me, the key was to remain as physically and mentally active as possible. Despite being confused over some words, letters, and numbers (even my wife's name), I confronted them over and over until they began making sense. I refused to just give in and wait until I was off chemotherapy. I had to fight back; it's just who I am.

Fighting to concentrate was the same. Although I often read the same paragraph time and time again, I kept reading, sometimes pronouncing each word aloud until I felt as if I had made some progress. And I would eat cold grits and eggs, not as a punishment, but to remind me of the very thing that was happening.

The effects on my short-term memory were perhaps the most troublesome for me to accept. I wasn't sharp, and I couldn't respond to a question without digging through my mind for the answers. Sometimes the answer came, sometimes it didn't, and sometimes I simply forgot the question and had to start over again. And although I can multitask, I still like to do things my way: one item at a time.

My cognitive functioning is now as good as it was before the chemotherapy, except on those days when I have a chemo day. During this time, nausea, severe fatigue, cognitive impairment, and usually diarrhea do their best to control me. I still find that if I force myself out of bed and do as much as is mentally and physically possible, I seem to function better until I return to normal.

The neuropathy in my fingertips and toes began during my second chemotherapy treatment and then spread to my fingers and the front part of my feet. I describe the sensation as tingling, numbness, and/or burning. It subsided in my fingers within four months after my last chemotherapy treatment. However, the neuropathy in my feet still remains. I've talked with nutritionists, chiropractors, and physicians about how to relieve this side effect, but no one seems to have an answer. Well, they all have answers, but nothing that can tell me when the discomfort will end. The Internet is loaded with would-be cures, and I've tried a few, including foot patches, but as of this writing nothing has worked for me. One company even advertised lab results from the black residue left on a patch after I had used it according to their recommendations if I sent it to them in a pre-labeled envelope that was part of the original box I purchased at a health food store. Was the residue from my foot, or a reaction from the chemicals? I have no idea. I never heard back from the company.

The cramping in my cheeks whenever I ate began during my first chemotherapy treatment. This side effect subsided within the first month after I had completed chemotherapy. I've only had it return twice during a chemo day.

The side effect of diarrhea was embarrassing and kept me close to home while undergoing chemotherapy. It ended shortly after the last treatment, but still coexists with nausea a couple of times a month.

The redness or flushing in my face began during my third chemotherapy treatment and was very pronounced during the first week of treatment. It also accompanies every chemo day. It is still with me in late afternoons and evenings, but by the following morning, my color returns to normal.

The metallic taste in my mouth disappeared within a month after the last chemotherapy treatment, but it does resurface during my occasional chemo day. In fact, it appears to be the first of the side effects to introduce a new chemo day.

My taste buds, which left for a long holiday when I underwent chemotherapy, appear to be home for good, along with a healthy appetite. It seems as though they are back with intensity. The taste of food is better than I remembered. Meats have better flavor, vegetables have a more distinct taste, and fruits are sweeter.

My hair thinned during chemotherapy, especially on the top. New hair did grow back, but not as much as I had before. I was one of the lucky ones who didn't go bald, but baldness has a beauty of its own.

During the third chemotherapy treatment, my skin felt as though no-see-ums were crawling all over me. A back scratcher helped, and after my last chemotherapy session, the itching gradually diminished to a level I could handle—perhaps equal to a number five on the smiley face pain chart in the hospital. (Though at times I feel as though the no-see-ums are back, especially during a chemo day.)

I've also had dental problems: more cavities, caps, a root canal, and gum problems. The number of visits to my dentist has more than tripled since finishing chemotherapy. "Not related," Dr. Rosen said last year during my yearly checkup. But the fact is that my dentist recommended no dental work while receiving chemotherapy—not even for a cleaning because of the increased possibility of infection. After talking to other chemotherapy survivors and researching the Internet, chemotherapy does play a significant role in tooth decay and oral problems during and after treatment. This information is not from a site controlled by the medical profession, rather from a site for comments from those individuals with increased dental problems after chemotherapy and radiation. My advice, while undergoing chemotherapy and/or radiation, is to brush your teeth after every meal, before you go to bed, and when you first wake in the morning. Otherwise, there isn't much more that can be done while receiving chemotherapy and/ or radiation. (I also use "brush picks" two to three times daily to remove food that could be trapped between my teeth.)

Against my physician's recommendation, I chose to have the Portacath removed after my last chemotherapy treatment. I know several cancer and chemotherapy survivors who elected to keep the Portacath after their last treatment. They seem to be unaware that there is still a bump under their skin, except when they take a shower and look at themselves in the mirror. "It's just a way of life," one woman said. "And it's there if I need it again."

I'm not advising anyone to follow my decision. Listen to your physician and make your own choice. For me, leaving the Portacath in my chest and feeling the bump every day when I showered would be a reminder much worse than daily viewing the scar where it once was. I believe that negative thoughts beget negative results. To me, keeping the Portacath inside my chest was like saying, "When the cancer does return, I'll be ready for it." It's almost as if I were inviting it back.

I also believe that positive thoughts beget positive results. So there was only one real choice for me. Take it out. By not seeing it, feeling it inside me, or touching it, I was making the statement that I will continue to fight my nemesis with every ounce of my energy. I was saying that cancer was not welcome here.

Fear of the unknown can be overwhelming. But when faced with cancer and chemotherapy and/or radiation, or any other disease or life challenge, once we commit to fight with every ounce or our total beings, I believe courage surfaces from within that enables us to combat anything we face. I now realize that fear exists only when we try to imagine the future. It's natural to want to know what is ahead;

whether it's waiting for test results from a colonoscopy or speculating about surgery, the effects of chemotherapy and/or radiation, or the continuing side effects that accompany an unknown chemo day or the anticipation of the five-year date for surviving cancer that a physician uses as the benchmark for survival. But if we know what is coming, it can ease the burden of the unknown and make the life challenge we face more manageable.

Do not withdraw from life if you have cancer; embrace it and enlist all those who are willing to help. There is good in everyone. Sickness is just one denominator that helps it surface. However, there could be friends who will be lost—were they really friends? But others will emerge with love and kindness that will amaze you.

Cancer does suck, but so does every sickness and disease known to mankind. I believe that the good in this world trumps evil tenfold, and I seek to find the goodness of all life wherever I go. There is nothing greater than the love we receive from others, or the love we give to others.

I will fight cancer with every good cell in my body. I will do my best to alleviate negativity from my thoughts. I will never give up. Never! And I hope you will do the same.